Clinical Point Selection

by the same author

Taoist Nei Dan Inner Meditation
An Accessible Guide
David Twicken
ISBN 978 1 83997 387 1
eISBN 978 1 83997 388 8

The Divergent Channels - Jing Bie
A Handbook for Clinical Practice and Five Shen Nei Dan Inner Meditation
Dr David Twicken DOM, LAc
ISBN 978 1 84819 189 1
eISBN 978 0 85701 150 3

Eight Extraordinary Channels - Qi Jing Ba Mai
A Handbook for Clinical Practice and Nei Dan Inner Meditation
Dr David Twicken DOM, LAc
ISBN 978 1 84819 148 8
eISBN 978 0 85701 137 4

The Luo Collaterals
A Handbook for Clinical Practice and Treating Emotions
and the Shen and The Six Healing Sounds
Dr David Twicken DOM, LAc
ISBN 978 1 84819 230 0
eISBN 978 0 85701 219 7

I Ching Acupuncture - The Balance Method
Clinical Applications of the Ba Gua and I Ching
Dr David Twicken DOM, LAc
ISBN 9781848190740
9780857010643

of related interest

Experiencing Acupuncture
Journeys of Body, Mind and Spirit for Patients and Practitioners
John Hamwee
ISBN 978 1 78775 250 4
eISBN 978 1 78775 251 1

The Beginner's Guide to the Eight Extraordinary Vessels
Mikschal (Dolma) Johanison D.Ac., L.Ac.
ISBN 978 1 78775 831 5
eISBN 978 1 78775 832 2

Applying Stems and Branches Acupuncture in Clinical Practice
Dynamic Dualities in Classical Chinese Medicine
Joan Duveen
Foreword by Tae Hunn Lee
ISBN 978 1 78775 370 9
eISBN 978 1 78775 371 6

CLINICAL POINT SELECTION

Classical, Traditional and Twicken Style Acupuncture

David Twicken

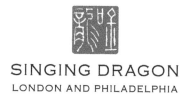

SINGING DRAGON
LONDON AND PHILADELPHIA

First published in Great Britain in 2025 by Singing Dragon,
an imprint of Jessica Kingsley Publishers
Part of John Murray Press

1

Copyright © David Twicken 2025

The right of David Twicken to be identified as the Author of the Work has been
asserted by him in accordance with the Copyright, Designs and Patents Act 1988.

Front cover image source: Depositphotos.com

All rights reserved. No part of this publication may be reproduced, stored
in a retrieval system, or transmitted, in any form or by any means without
the prior written permission of the publisher, nor be otherwise circulated
in any form of binding or cover other than that in which it is published and
without a similar condition being imposed on the subsequent purchaser.

A CIP catalogue record for this title is available from the
British Library and the Library of Congress

ISBN 978 1 80501 206 1
eISBN 978 1 80501 207 8

Printed and bound in the United States by Integrated Books International

Jessica Kingsley Publishers' policy is to use papers that are natural,
renewable and recyclable products and made from wood grown in
sustainable forests. The logging and manufacturing processes are expected
to conform to the environmental regulations of the country of origin.

Singing Dragon
Carmelite House
50 Victoria Embankment
London EC4Y 0DZ

www.singingdragon.com

John Murray Press
Part of Hodder & Stoughton Limited
An Hachette UK Company

The authorised representative in the EEA is Hachette Ireland, 8 Castlecourt
Centre, Castleknock Road, Castleknock, Dublin 15, D15 YF6A, Ireland

Disclaimer

The information in this book is based on the author's knowledge and personal experience. This information is presented for educational purposes to assist the reader in expanding his or her knowledge of Chinese philosophy and Chinese medicine. The techniques and practices are to be used at the reader's own discretion and liability. The author is not responsible in any manner whatsoever for any physical injury that may occur by following instructions in this book. Consult a licensed healthcare practitioner for medical treatment.

Contents

 Author's Note. 9

 About This Book 11

 Introduction. 17

1. What Is Acupuncture? 21
2. How Acupuncture Works 31
3. Working within Channels. 37
4. Reinforcing and Reducing Channels. 47
5. The Conduit Vessels: The Main Channels 55
6. Channel Selection. 59
7. Acupuncture Point Categories in the Han Dynasty . . . 67
8. Treating Organs. 83
9. Treating Emotions 97
10. Treating Pain 111
11. Professional Reviews 123

 Conclusion. 163

 Bibliography 165

 Index. 167

Author's Note

During the long history of Chinese medicine, many traditions and methods for the practice of acupuncture have developed. Practitioners may apply approaches in this book along with their existing methods practiced or they may choose to use the approaches in this book as a stand-alone system. The theories and applications in this book are flexible and can be applied in any clinical setting.

The following are explanations for some terms used in this book.

Imbalance means any pathological pathogen and condition, which includes the six exogenous factors, seven endogenous factors, Qi stagnation, blood stagnation and deficiencies and excesses of the internal organs. Imbalance is a general term used to describe any unfavorable conditions in the body. All conditions can be filtered into an excess, deficiency or a combination of the two.

Acupuncture point means the specific acupuncture points listed in modern acupuncture books, as well as any areas of treatment, which can be non-acupuncture points. The non-acupuncture points include ashi areas and anatomical imaging areas that can be treated. An acupuncture point is any area that is treated; this is a broad definition for any area treated.

The *reinforcing and reducing* technique is how a device is manipulated. It is a technique that can be applied to any acupuncture point or area on the body. This is not an acupuncture point that is labeled as a reinforcing or reducing acupuncture point—for example, lung 9 is a reinforcing point in five-phases theory as it is the earth point on the metal channel, the lung. In *Nan Ching* five-phases theory, earth is the parent phase of the metal/Lung channel. It is the five-phases reinforcing acupuncture point, it is not a needling technique. The needling technique can be applied to any area on the body. A five-phases parent point is a theory. Reinforcing needling is a technique, a physical method of manipulation to create an internal reaction (movement).

Reinforcing means to move Qi (bio-electricity) to an area, which can be an organ, a gland or an area of the body—for example, moving Qi to the Spleen, Liver or Kidney to reinforce them. From an acupuncture viewpoint, reinforcing, supplementing, tonifying, fortifying and nourishing mean the same thing: to move Qi to the area/organ to bring it into balance (a normal condition or the level of restoration that is possible).

Reducing means to remove, clear, drain, break down or move the condition to allow it to be resolved with the treatment or with the body's natural processes. From an acupuncture viewpoint, reducing, sedating and clearing mean the same thing.

The words *channels*, *meridians* and *pathways* are used interchangeably. Channels include the physiology of the channel system, which is explained throughout the book.

Qi includes the function of bio-electricity.

About This Book

Clinical Point Selection is my fifth book on Chinese medicine. Two of the main focuses of this book are examining areas of ambiguity regarding acupuncture point selection found in common texts and teachings, and offering a systematic approach to creating acupuncture treatments that brings clarity in theory and application. This book includes an explanation of how acupuncture works from an acupuncture channel perspective, which becomes the basis for creating acupuncture treatments. The acupuncture theories, strategies and methods presented in this book are rooted in acupuncture classics and traditional Chinese medicine (TCM), and they are expanded and clarified in key ways by my insights of integrating classical theories not commonly presented as an integrated system. This book primarily contains approaches to create acupuncture treatments using the twelve main channels but include the sinew, luo, divergent and the Eight Extraordinary Channels. For more detailed information on those channels see my books *Eight Extraordinary Channels*, *The Luo Collaterals*, *The Divergent Channels,* and *I Ching Acupuncture—The Balance Method*.

Clinical point selection in classical and traditional acupuncture includes a systematic approach to developing acupuncture treatments for clinical practice. This channel-based acupuncture system presented in this book integrates foundational acupuncture theories found in classical, traditional and modern texts and my insights, which are the basis for a logical, systematic framework to create acupuncture treatments. The organization

CLINICAL POINT SELECTION

and guiding principles of each step in the selection of channels, acupuncture points and areas to be treated are what make this a system. This system utilizes the channels, acupuncture points, techniques and modalities learned at Chinese medical schools; there are no new channels or acupuncture points in this acupuncture treatment approach. I have identified and clearly explained aspects of acupuncture point selection and treatment that aren't discussed or are vague in texts and textbooks, bringing clarity and intention to clinical practice.

It was surprising to me that there are no case studies or examples of how to develop a complete acupuncture plan and its implementation in *Nei Jing Su Wen*, *Jia Yi Jing* and other early classics. This exclusion leads the practitioner to create whatever they think may be effective or to follow what others present. This book is my effort to bring this area of vagueness to the forefront of our profession with the hope that more practitioners will contribute their clinical experiences and elevate our level of education and practice. The channel-based method in this book is a classical and traditional acupuncture approach that can remove the vagueness and ambiguity in creating acupuncture treatments.

Clinical Point Selection presents a channel-based acupuncture approach which includes three main components:

1. Treatments are applied in the channel system presented in the Han dynasty. It is the skill of the practitioner to influence the body via the channel system that creates the therapeutic effect (clinical effectiveness).

2. Treatments include a reinforcing or reducing strategy. That strategy includes a needling technique and the needling sequence of the acupuncture points—that is, areas treated.

3. Treatments include directionality, which includes the reinforcing or reducing strategy and the use of destination acupuncture points. The reinforcing and reducing needling method contributes to the directionality of the treatment.

The following list contains the basic steps a practitioner should include when creating and applying channel-based acupuncture treatments. Each of the three main parts of clinical practice listed above and the steps listed below are presented and explained throughout this book.

1. Identify the imbalanced channels, organs and areas when developing a treatment plan. Chapter 3 of the *Ling Shu*, "Explanatory Remarks on the Small Needle," includes the following guidance: "First know which channels are diseased, then treat them at those locations."[1]

2. Determine whether the condition is excess or deficient.

3. Determine whether to apply a reinforcing or reducing technique; applying these techniques is essential in treatment. Chapter 1 of the *Ling Shu*, "The Nine Needles and the Twelve Source Points," states, "All use of acupuncture is thus: Tonify hollowness, disperse fullness."[2]

4. Decide on the acupuncture points and areas to be treated. Treating multiple acupuncture points is usually required to obtain the therapeutic effect. A synergy is created by multiple stimulations on a channel that no one point can generate. Strategically selecting areas for treatment to create the required circulation (movement) in the channels is the key to clinical effectiveness. It's all about creating movement in the channels and areas, which includes the directionality of the treatment plan.

5. Select the corresponding device for treatment; this is a key in clinical effectiveness, and includes the type of device—lancet, needle, needle length and gage, and so on. This aspect of treatment is essential for clinical efficacy.

---

[1] Wu, J. (2002) *Ling Shu or The Spiritual Pivot*. Hawaii: University of Hawaii Press.
[2] Ibid.

6. Determine the needling sequence. This should be based on whether the treatment is reinforcing or reducing. Including needle sequencing is a central aspect of this channel-based system. Applying this approach is one of the most significant aspects of the reinforcing and reducing method. Follow the treatment sequence that corresponds to the needling technique. Needling sequence is explained in detail in this book.

7. Include destination points™ (the targeted areas in treatments). This is a crucial aspect of this approach to acupuncture treatment; it significantly increases clinical effectiveness.

8. Determine if the treatment requires supporting channels. The Yin-Yang paired channel should be the first supporting channel considered; those paired channels connect to each other's organ, therefore can treat each other. Additional channels to be considered include the six-channel paired channel and channels with internal pathways that intersect with the channel, organ or areas of imbalance.

9. Include whether there should be stimulation during the treatment. This includes a timeframe to check the patient's response to the treatment—for example, checking on the patient every 10, 15 or 20 minutes. Checking the pulse is one classical method to determine if more stimulation or treatment time is necessary. Dosage and duration are key in acupuncture treatments. The dosage is the number of points and the intensity of stimulation, along with the duration of the treatment.

10. Include the effectiveness test™ as this significantly increases efficiency and effectiveness when treating pain. The chapter "Treating Pain" in this book introduces the effectiveness test.

11. Include the appropriate Chinese medical modalities for each treatment: bodywork, moxibustion, cupping, liniments and Chinese herbs.

Including the steps listed comprises a systematic approach to developing treatments. I have organized the main elements of treatments from classical and traditional Chinese medicine as well as my insights into a logical order that creates a treatment synergy. Each aspect of the treatment increases the synergistic effect, requiring less manual stimulation on each area since multiple stimulations combine to become one targeted influence to achieve the therapeutic effect. This targeted influence will be clearly explained throughout the text. A comprehensive understanding of the relationships and connections that exist in an integrated channel-based system allows the practitioner to create treatments that are precise, efficient and effective—they are customized treatments.

Introduction

The earliest Chinese medical manuscripts are from the Warring States period of the Zhou dynasty (403–221 BCE). These manuscripts, known as the *Mawangdui Silk Texts*, were found buried in the tomb of a member of the royal family from the Han dynasty (206 BCE–220 CE). The tomb was sealed in 163 BCE. The manuscripts were discovered in the Hunan Province in 1973.

The *Mawangdui* manuscripts discuss three main treatment methods: herbal, bloodletting and moxibustion (moxa). Moxa is the burning of the herb mugwort (*Artemisiae argyi* folium) and other herbs and substances over and on the body. Bloodletting is pricking areas of the body to cause bleeding, which allows pathogens in the blood to be removed from the body.

The *Mawangdui* manuscripts describe pathways that flow throughout the body. The pathways are not as detailed nor do they have the same internal organ intersections as found in *Nei Jing Ling Shu* and *Su Wen*. They do reflect early Chinese medical insight about pathways. It is important to note that there are no acupuncture points or acupuncture techniques in the *Mawangdui* manuscripts.

The Han dynasty acupuncture classic *Nei Jing Ling Shu* includes about 160 acupuncture points. The text presents a variety of needles and needling techniques. Below are eight key additions that the *Nei Jing Ling Shu* made to Chinese medicine:

CLINICAL POINT SELECTION

1. New channels that comprise a channel system: the tendo-muscle channels, the luo collaterals, the divergent channels and the Eight Extraordinary Channels.
2. More detailed channel trajectories.
3. Yin-Yang organ and channel theory, including that each of the twelve channels intersects with its own organ and its Yin-Yang paired organ.
4. Approximately 160 acupuncture points.
5. Acupuncture point categories.
6. Channel treatments.
7. Acupuncture point treatments.
8. Needling devices and needling techniques.

The *Nei Jing Ling Shu* includes both channel and acupuncture point treatment theories and applications. From a historical viewpoint, it is clear that channel theory and treatment occurred first, and the individual acupuncture points appeared later. Understanding the relationship between channels and acupuncture points is essential in applying acupuncture in an effective way. *Nei Jing* presents two main ways to treat an imbalance. The first is to treat areas on the channels and the second is to treat acupuncture points that treat specific indications (based on symptoms, the acupuncture points can be from any channel). Chapter 64 of the *Ling Shu*, "The Yin and Yang and the 25 Human Types," presents a way to determine areas to select for treatment on pathways:

> One touches the inch opening and renying [opening] to balance yin and yang. One presses the fingers along the conduits and network [vessels] until they have reached [a section that is] rough with lumps. Where there are knots blocking the passage, this will result in a blockage-illness all over the body. In serious cases the movement is stopped, and this results in [sections that are] rough

with lumps. [Sections that are] rough with lumps can be ended by warming the qi and harmonizing the blood. As for knotted network [vessels], the vessels are knotted and the blood is not in harmony. When that is resolved the movement can continue.[1]

The quote above guides the practitioner to identify the imbalanced channel by taking the pulse, in this case the Renying-Cunkou pulse (any diagnostic method can be used to identify the imbalanced channel) and then to inspect the entire channel, from beginning to end, to locate the places of imbalances and then treat them directly. The use of both traditional acupuncture points and areas on a channel should be included in treatment strategies and clinical point selection.

---

[1] Unschuld, P. (2016) *Huang Di Nei Jing Ling Shu: The Ancient Classic on Needle Therapy*. University of California Press.

CHAPTER 1

What Is Acupuncture?

Acupuncture is a method to treat areas of the body with devices (most commonly the filiform needle). The basic approach is to insert a needle (device) in an acupuncture point which is on an acupuncture channel. The device is manipulated to create a reaction within the body to achieve the desired clinical result. That combination—inserting a device into the body and then stimulating it—is the fundamental process of an acupuncture treatment. My experience is that the insertion and manipulation of the device is responsible for 50 percent or more of the effectiveness of the treatment; the acupuncture process only occurs when that action occurs. All the functions of acupuncture points in books can only occur when the needle is inserted and stimulated. The ability to stimulate the needle is the key to an effective treatment; that is a skill the practitioner needs to develop. Acupuncture is a skill-based healing system.

The acupuncture channel system

The *Ling Shu* is considered the primary Han dynasty source for the practice of acupuncture. The book includes a channel system called *Jing Luo*, which is a map of the human body and the terrain for treatment. Over the last 2000 years, theories have been overlaid on the channel system. Some theories are rooted in classical acupuncture theories, others are not. My intention in this book is to provide insight about the structure and function of the acupuncture channel system before the many theories were overlaid on the channels. Understanding the original structure and function of the channel system will free the practitioner from rigid theories, applications and prepackaged methods commonly taught, and it will allow for a clear and direct understanding and application for clinical point selection.

The structure of acupuncture channels

Acupuncture has a structure and function. Practitioners and scholars from the many traditions of acupuncture agree on the structure; in fact, it may be the most agreed-on area in the whole field of acupuncture. The structure is the channel system and its pathway network. Every professional acupuncture book from the *Nei Jing* to modern texts includes the channel system and its pathways. The channel system reveals the unique insight of the ancient Chinese medical practitioners, and it is where the acupuncture activity primarily occurs.

The function of the acupuncture channels

There are numerous acupuncture theories and applications in the practice of acupuncture. In this book, I propose that the movement of Qi and blood within the body—specifically the acupuncture channels—is the original function in the channels. It is more accurate to name channels with their original names: hand and foot Taiyang, Shaoyang and Yangming, and hand and foot Taiyin, Shaoyin and Jueyin. Using those names provides the understanding that the channels include the entire area where the channels flow, including the trajectory internally, and all the anatomy and physiology it flows to, as well as where the points are located. Treatments can influence the entire trajectory, not just an organ.

And treatment not only moves Qi and blood, but the entire channel physiology, which moves the Qi and blood inside it. *This is a key mechanism to understand*—the ability to move the entire channel anatomy and physiology leads to increased clinical effectiveness. Having a comprehensive understanding of what a channel is leads to more efficient and effective acupuncture treatments. The classics imply a comprehensive understanding of a channel but it is not clearly presented. Wang Ju-Yi, in his book *Applied Channel Theory in Chinese Medicine*, presents some insightful descriptions of a channel.

> The channel system connects the internal organs to one another, to the surface of the body, and to the environment at large. The channel network unifies the other systems of the body—digestive, lymphatic, nervous, reproductive, and others into a coherent and responsive whole.[1]

> Again, it is important to remember that the network of channels is itself an integral part of physiology in classical Chinese medicine. In other words, the channels are "alive" in the same way that one might consider the heart or lung to be alive.[2]

> They act as pathways not only for the flow of substances like interstitial fluids *around* these anatomical structures, but also for the flow *within* the structures.[3]

> As one might surmise, not only do these pathways conduct the elements of a healthy physiology, they also serve as conduits for disease.[4]

Treating the internal organs is a main modern application of the primary channels. The classical treatment method is needling. This book focuses on clinical point selection for the main channels.

[1] Wang, J. & Robertson, J. (2008) *Applied Channel Theory in Chinese Medicine: Wang Ju-Yi's Lectures on Channel Therapeutics.* Seattle, WA: Eastland Press.
[2] Ibid.
[3] Ibid.
[4] Ibid.

Having a comprehensive understanding of the structure and function of the channels guides the practitioner in how to best influence them to achieve treatment effectiveness.

Movement in the channels

The practitioner influences movement in the channel system with the combination of the channels and points treated, the needling sequence and the needling technique. The movement in the channels is either inward and toward an area, or outward, downward and away from an area. The reinforcing and reducing needling techniques determine those movements. The classics do not clearly state but imply that the entire channel, which includes the internal pathway, the structures it connects with, including the internal organs, glands, muscles, tendons and bones, and the main channel area, are all affected in treatment. The entire channel moves, which includes Qi and blood. The ability to move the entire channel is a key in clinical efficacy. The original name of the channels contains the names of the six channels—Taiyang, Shaoyang, Yangming, Taiyin, Shaoyin and Jueyin—and includes the entire channel and all its connections. Channels include much more than the associated organ.

Systems of correspondences and function

The systems of correspondences form one of the most important principles in Chinese philosophy and Chinese medicine—the understanding that things relate to and influence each other. That interactive relationship comprises a connection that can be stimulated to influence one or more of the parts of the correspondences. The early classic texts of Chinese medicine—*Su Wen*, *Ling Shu*, *Nan Ching* and *Jia Yi Jing*—include the most primary systems of correspondences: Yin-Yang and the five phases. Those two correspondences are the initial theories laid on top of the channels. *It is important to understand that Yin-Yang and the five phases are diagnostic models that identify imbalances within the channels and organs; they are not substances for treatment.* Qi (bio-electricity) is the primary substance influenced in the practice of acupuncture, and it is part of the original structure and function of the acupuncture channels. The ability of the practitioner to influence the body by stimulating the acupuncture channels and the Qi in them creates the therapeutic effect (the healing effect), which is the primary focus of treatment and this book.

The distribution of *Nei Jing*'s channel system can be viewed from superficial to deep layers of the body. The channel system includes the tendo-muscle channels, luo collaterals, primary channels, divergent channels and Eight Extraordinary Channels. Each of the channels has a unique relationship with layers of the body, pathogenic factors, vital substances and anatomical structures. Treating imbalances within the channel system to which they correspond increases clinical efficacy, and applying the corresponding treatment modality for each channel system increases clinical effectiveness. Treating the corresponding channel system and applying the corresponding treatment modalities is a unique insight of the ancient healers.

Nei Jing channel system (Jing Luo)

The sinew channels

The sinew channels are commonly known as the tendo-muscle channels; this channel system is presented in Chapter 13 of the *Ling Shu*, "The Muscle Channels or The Conduits and their Sinews." This channel system is the most superficial of the channels listed in this book. The chapter lists the signs, symptoms and conditions that correspond to the channels. *Ling Shu* guidance is to use a hot needle for treatment (warming the needle with fire) and to treat the painful areas directly, which is a local treatment. It also states that each channel corresponds to a specific month of the year and that there can be imbalances of each channel during its associated month.

The sinew channels are used for musculoskeletal conditions, of which pain is the main symptom. *Tui Na* (bodywork), acupuncture, moxa, cupping, liniments and treating ashi points are traditional modalities. Electroacupuncture is a modern healing modality. Placing moxa on a needle is an alternative for a hot needle. Orthopedic adjustments (chiropractic adjustments) are part of classical *Tui Na* training in China.

The luo collaterals

The luo collaterals are primarily presented in Chapter 10 of the *Ling Shu*, "The Main Channels." They are also discussed in numerous chapters in *Su Wen* and *Ling Shu*. The treatment method for the luo collaterals is bleeding the luo point or along the luo collateral.

Nei Jing states that the luo collaterals can be seen while the primary channels cannot, and the luo collaterals have no pulse while the primary channels have a pulse. The luo collaterals also have colors and specific pathogenic factors. Visual inspection of the luo is a key to diagnosis. The *Ling Shu* organizes signs and symptoms into deficiency and excess conditions. These collaterals are presented as buffers to hold pathogenic factors to prevent them from flowing deeper into the body. Pricking (bloodletting) is used to release the pathogens from the body. The luo collaterals are located at the superficial layer of the body, and the treatment method in turn treats the superficial layer. The *Nei Jing* clearly states that the luo collaterals do not treat the deep layers in the body, which includes the internal organs.

The classical treatment method is to bleed the luo point and the luo collateral.

The clinical theory and function of the luo collaterals has changed over time, based on a series of hypotheses. I present two common theories in Chapter 11 in this book. One review is about the luo collaterals and includes the history of the collaterals and new theories added which do not contain any supporting explanation of the theory. On reading the chapter, a practitioner can make an educated decision about how to use the luo collaterals in clinical practice.

The main channels

The main channels (commonly referred to as the primary channels) are introduced in Chapter 10 of the *Ling Shu*, "The Conduit Vessels." These channels are referenced in many chapters throughout *Su Wen* and *Ling Shu*. The main channels have become the central channel system used in modern TCM. The conditions listed in Chapter 10 of the *Ling Shu* and in other chapters contribute to making a diagnosis that includes a differential diagnosis of the internal organ systems.

Understanding the difference between an acupuncture point and a channel

There are two main ways to approach selecting acupuncture points. The first is symptomatic, which is usually presented as indications in acupuncture books. The second is a channel-based approach. The first states that each point treats a condition; the second approach includes the first but is not locked to one point treating the condition—any of the points or areas on a channel has the potential to treat any condition of an organ and channel. How is that possible? Acupuncture influences the entire channel to cause a reinforcing or reducing movement to treat the condition. It's the whole channel movement that creates the reinforcing or reducing movement. Every condition can be identified as excess or deficient, and is reinforced or reduced; it does not matter what the imbalance is (the modality can change from acupuncture needling to bloodletting, cupping, gua sha, etc.) as the movement in the channel creates the effective action. Five-phases acupuncture includes this reality—for an excess, treat the child acupuncture point; it will treat any excess, there is no differential diagnosis. The assumption is that the child reduces the channel better than any other point. The well points are another example, as they treat any conditions of the channels and organs from a *Nei Jing* viewpoint; it's the needling technique that determines if it's a reinforcing or reducing treatment. The *Nei Jing* and *Nan Ching* clearly state that the source points treat any conditions of the organs, and they are not limited to a particular pathogen or pattern. However, some teachers and practitioners will create narrow and rigid clinical applications of channels and acupuncture points. It's very important to know that difference; this book focuses on presenting that difference, which can open the possibilities for creating acupuncture treatments.

The key to creating effective acupuncture treatments is to stimulate the areas of a channel to achieve the clinical result. This book includes a wide approach for accomplishing that objective.

The divergent channels

The divergent channels are presented in Chapter 11 of the *Ling Shu*, "The Conduits and their Diverging [Vessels]." The divergent channels do not have acupuncture points; the pathways simply begin and end at the lower and upper areas of the body. The Yin and Yang primary channel pairs meet together via the divergent pathways to form a junction, which is classically named a *confluence*. The divergent channels chapter does not present any clinical applications. There is special guidance in the first paragraph of the chapter that can guide a practitioner to exploring clinical applications:

> Study these first. Work it out to the finish. The unskilled think it is easy; the superior know it is difficult. Please explain these separations and joinings, these exits and entrance. How illuminating are these questions. The skilled pass right by them, while they are the very breath of the superior physician.[5]

After that guidance, the pathways of the divergent channels are

---

5 Wu, J. (2002) *Ling Shu or The Spiritual Pivot.* Hawaii: University of Hawaii Press.

presented. A practical application of this guidance would be to integrate theories and applications in the chapters in the *Ling Shu* and *Su Wen* to these channels. My approach includes using the divergent channels to treat conditions along their pathways as well as to use them to support their Yin-Yang paired channel and corresponding channel systems. For example, the bladder divergent channel flows along the spine, and the Du channel also flows on the spine. The bladder divergent channel can support a Du channel treatment because it flows in the same area as the Du channel (a spine treatment). Any theory and clinical application of the divergent channels should be critically evaluated, as it is someone's view that is not presented in *Nei Jing* and other acupuncture texts.

There is no treatment method for the divergent channels in the classics. See my book *The Divergent Channels—Jing Bie* for more information on how to apply them in clinical practice.

The Eight Extraordinary Vessels (EVs)

Information on the eight EVs is found throughout the *Su Wen* and *Ling Shu*, including Chapters 16, 17, 21, 23, 38, 62, 65 and 80 in the *Ling Shu* and Chapters 39, 59, 60, and 63 in *Su Wen*. The EVs are not presented as a comprehensive system in any one chapter. In most cases, EV points are listed with conditions they treat in a symptomatic way. It is important to note that there are no pathway descriptions for the Yang and Yin Wei channels; it would not be possible to do a Yin Wei or Yang Wei treatment based on *Su Wen* and *Ling Shu*. There does not seem to be a clear history and reasoning of who determined the Yin and Yang Wei pathway descriptions and their points. The points are listed in more modern versions of the *Jia Yi Jing* (*Classic of Acupuncture and Moxibustion* by Huang-fu Mi). It is said the *Jia Yi Jing* was first published in 282 CE. The earliest version available is from the Ming dynasty, 1601 CE.[6]

---

6 Yang, C. (2004) *A Systematic Classic of Acupuncture and Moxibustion*. Boulder, CO: Blue Poppy Press.

The EVs can be applied in clinical practice based on the specific conditions and functions found in the *Su Wen* and *Ling Shu* or from theories added over the past 2000 years. The new theories and applications should be evaluated to determine their relevancy to Chinese medicine. In this book, I present a major hypothesis that changed the way these channels are used in treatments. It's a hypothesis I do not follow as I see no way it can be effective based on any classical acupuncture theories. I present a professional review of the Eight Intersection Points of the Eight Extraordinary Channels in this book; they are commonly referred to as the opening, command, master or confluent points of the Eight Extraordinary Channels (Vessels).

Su Wen and *Ling Shu* practitioners provided a road map of the human body that includes five main channel systems to be used in clinical practice. Their vision provided a profound understanding of the correspondences between areas of the body, acupuncture channels, pathogenic factors and treatment methods, and within their insight is the understanding that each channel system most effectively treats imbalances in its corresponding areas of the body. Treating the right channel system with the right treatment modality is the key to clinical effectiveness—that is the essential guidance found in *Su Wen* and *Ling Shu*.

CHAPTER 2

How Acupuncture Works

Modern researchers and practitioners seek to find the mechanisms for how acupuncture works from a biomedical viewpoint. However, this has not revealed a definitive understanding of how it works. The tools of modern medicine identify that acupuncture has an effect—for example, imaging can show how inflammation decreases with acupuncture treatment. It is my experience as a practitioner, teacher and supervisor of interns at acupuncture schools that acupuncture functions within the acupuncture channels and the key to clinical efficacy is the ability of the practitioner to influence targeted aspects of the channels.

Models of Chinese Medicine

Yin-Yang, five phases, six channels, zangfu and the herbalization of acupuncture points are main models used in classical and traditional acupuncture. Those models organize conditions and this then provides the basis for diagnosis and a treatment plan. These models are theoretical layers on top of the original activity in the channels: acupuncture stimulates movement in the channels to a targeted area (reinforcement) or out and away (reducing). These movements are the natural way the body functions, and when there is an imbalance where normal movement is altered, it can lead to illness. This original movement is within all the models of acupuncture, and how movement can be adjusted can vary with each model.

Models have strengths and weaknesses. Models organize information, provide a focus on understanding a health condition and suggest options for treatment. The process of organizing conditions can limit what is actually occurring as the model forces all conditions into a rigid framework. That forcing can remove an essential aspect of classical and traditional acupuncture—customizing treatments for each individual person. That customization approach is the widest application of diagnosis and treatment, meaning it is not forced into a model with fixed treatments. Being able to navigate through the common models of acupuncture and the original understanding of movement allows us to understand, work with and optimize the use of the models of acupuncture. The original activity of acupuncture is presented throughout the book.

Each channel has a precise trajectory that flows throughout the body. When a practitioner stimulates one area of the trajectory, that stimulation can influence anywhere along the channel. The trajectory can be stimulated to influence a targeted area, or it can be stimulated to cause an outward and away movement. It is either a reinforcing or reducing acupuncture technique that directs those actions. It is commonly presented that when a reinforcing or reducing technique is applied, the Qi inside the channel system moves to cause a directional reaction: this is the activity in the acupuncture channels. To be more precise, the entire channel moves and the substances inside it move too. From a classical acupuncture viewpoint, a channel is alive in the same way the internal organs are alive. The channel is part of the body's physiology, including the internal organs, glands, bones, muscles, tendons and skin—they are all one inseparable whole. The practitioner can strategically stimulate any aspect of a channel with the proper device, acupuncture points sequence, needle depth and stimulation method.

The reinforcing or reducing acupuncture technique and the

needle sequence are the *adjusting method* for creating directionality and location in treatment. The needling sequence combined with the needling technique and destination points (local points) more precisely determines the direction and location of a treatment.

Needling sequence

The needling sequence participates in creating the direction in treatment and is essential in a treatment plan but is not mentioned in common teachings regarding acupuncture. In my experience, direction is one of the most important aspects of a treatment. Practicing nei dan internal meditation led me to understand how to incorporate directionality into acupuncture treatments (see Chapter 3 for information on nei dan internal meditation). One of the most important and influential actions a practitioner can include in their practice is needle sequencing. For example, it is common to select Spleen 3, the source point, to reinforce the Spleen. The practitioner needles Spleen 3, preferably with a reinforcing technique. The hope is that needling Spleen 3 will cause Qi in the Spleen channel to move into the Spleen. My experience is that using a single point is often not effective. If Spleen 9 is added, there is a stronger force than needling only one point. It is hoped that the two points and their collective influence move enough Qi within the channel to fill the Spleen with Qi and restore it to its normal function. Two is better than one in most cases.

The order is important. If the goal is to reinforce the Spleen by stimulating the Spleen channel, causing movement up the channel into the Spleen, the two points on the Spleen channel need to create a movement/vibration/stimulation that is stronger than needling one point. It is much more effective to begin at the most distal area and then move closer to the area in which the treatment is being directed; the needling sequence is distal to local. In this case, needling Spleen 3 and then Spleen 9 is most effective. Additionally, it is generally more effective to needle up one side of the channel to create a stronger influence (movement) than treating the right side of the body and then the left side, which alters the momentum up the channel. The method would be to needle left Spleen 6 and left Spleen 9 and then right Spleen 6 and right Spleen 9. The ipsilateral order is essential in creating a stronger therapeutic effect (moment) within the channel; it generates stronger movement into the Spleen. The ipsilateral needle sequence should be the guiding principle for most treatments. Applying other methods should be the exception and should be guided by a specific strategy.

The therapeutic effect

A treatment plan includes the degree of stimulation required to obtain the desired healing result. In herbal medicine, prescribing the effective dosage is necessary to obtain the desired effect. The same is true in acupuncture: applying the correct dosage is key in clinical efficacy. Dosage in acupuncture includes the number of channels/points/areas to be treated, the sequence in which the needles are inserted, the reinforcing/reducing technique and the frequency and degree of stimulation of the needles. Unlike herbal medicine, acupuncture has methods that quickly measure the effectiveness of the treatment, and these include pulse diagnosis, palpation, visual inspection and questioning.

Channels and acupuncture points, unifying the great disconnect

Understanding the connection between internal pathways, anatomical areas, internal organs and acupuncture points is the first step in understanding how acupuncture works from a classical acupuncture theory viewpoint. For example, if a patient is Spleen Qi deficient and the treatment plan is to reinforce the Spleen, the goal is to select points on the Spleen channel to reinforce the Spleen. The question is, what occurs during a reinforcing treatment? The Spleen pathway flows from the well point—Spleen 1—up the channel to connect to the Spleen. The objective is to stimulate the Spleen channel to increase the degree to which Qi is already flowing up the channel into the Spleen. Stimulation is the key.

I use the term *therapeutic effect* to describe the effect of the treatment. A goal is to determine the amount of stimulation necessary to obtain the desired therapeutic effect; this can be viewed as the dosage. The primary objective is to understand how the treatment is influencing the channel and the targeted area; determining how many points need to be treated to obtain the therapeutic effect is crucial in treatment. This is not a point-driven approach; it is a channel-driven approach. The ability to stimulate the channel to obtain the desired therapeutic effect is the objective. This treatment style is guided by the understanding that acupuncture points, channels and their trajectories are one inseparable whole.

Measuring treatment effect

Chapter 9 of the *Ling Shu*, "From Beginning to End," guides the practitioner to periodically check the pulse after the needles are inserted to measure whether the treatment causes a change in the pulse; this is a measuring function. When the pulse changes toward a balanced state, the guidance is to remove the needles because the treatment has accomplished its goal. This pulse method is a way to measure treatment effectiveness, and the approach can be applied to other pulse systems. Developing an awareness of a patient's response to treatment is essential in attuning to the therapeutic effect; it allows for the practitioner to adjust treatment while with the patient. This is an essential aspect of classical Chinese medicine.

The activity created by an acupuncture treatment primarily

occurs within the acupuncture channels. It is the ability of the practitioner to influence the activity by selecting the appropriate number of points for treatment and applying the proper needling sequence and technique that directly influences clinical effectiveness. This channel-based system of treatment effectively influences the acupuncture activity to obtain a clinically effective therapeutic effect.

CHAPTER 3

Working within Channels

The *Ling Shu* provides essential guidance for creating a treatment plan: identify the imbalanced channel and location to treat, and then determine whether to reinforce or reduce. Chapter 3 of the *Ling Shu*, "Explanatory Remarks on the Small Needle," includes the following: "First know which channels are diseased, then treat them at those locations."[1] In addition, Chapter 1 of the *Ling Shu*, "The Nine Needles and the Twelve Origin [Openings]," states, "All use of acupuncture is thus: Tonify hollowness, disperse fullness."[2]

Reinforcing means to guide Qi to an area or location. Reducing means to guide pathogens out and away from an area. The purpose of an acupuncture treatment is to stimulate the body via the channels to achieve the therapeutic effect. The guidance for where to treat (the locations of the diseases) is clearly stated in the quote above.

Nei Jing reinforcing and reducing methods are found in a variety of chapters, including *Su Wen*, Chapter 27, "Pathogens" and Chapter 54, "The Art of Acupuncture," and *Ling Shu*, Chapter 1, "Nine Needles and Twelve Source Points. The Laws of Heaven" and Chapter 3, "An Explanation of the Minute Needles. The Laws of Man."

---

1   Wu, J. (2002) *Ling Shu or The Spiritual Pivot*. Hawaii: University of Hawaii Press.
2   Ibid.

Activity during treatment

There are two main insights that brought clarity and precision to my understanding of how acupuncture works. The first is the teachings of Dr. Chao Chen, founder of the Balance Method and I Ching acupuncture; the second is nei dan inner meditation.

Dr. Chen taught practitioners to directly treat imbalanced channels and organs, which follows the foundation of *Ling Shu* guidance: identify the imbalanced channel/organ and treat it directly. Additionally, Dr. Chen emphasized that a key to treatment effectiveness is creating movement (circulation) in the channels. He stressed that stimulating channels is the way to balance the imbalanced channel or organ, regardless of the specific condition; it is not pattern based. He did not believe that one point and only that point could treat the list of conditions seen in acupuncture books. A channel and its trajectory comprise one inseparable system, and it is the practitioner's skill that effectively applies the stimulus to generate the desired therapeutic effect in a channel.

Dr. Chen explained that the initial way to treat a channel (and anything along it) is to treat the stream and sea points. He claimed that acupuncture point combination is not about the specific qualities of each point, it is about effectively stimulating a channel to create circulation to achieve the desired therapeutic effect. The therapeutic-effect mechanism occurs in two ways:

1. Acupuncture channels are circuits the practitioner can influence by causing movement that clears blockages and restores the normal function of the channels, organs and areas along the channels. The clearing is reducing and the direction is outward, downward and away.

2. Increasing circulation (movement) in the channels can increase Qi (bio-electricity) flow within them to targeted areas to balance channels/organs. This is reinforcing and the direction is inward and toward an organ or area.

Circulation is the reason for the effectiveness of this method. Circulation, the number of areas of treatment, the needling sequence and the needling technique combine to create a moving force that is vital for effective treatment. That moving force is the precise influence that creates the healing effect. This approach has a broad influence; it can restore an organ and channel regardless of the specific signs, symptoms and internal organ patterns. One might ask, how can that happen? The following insights help explain this healing process.

Reinforcing and reducing needling technique creates movement

Here are some important modern viewpoints on how acupuncture works:

> Note that here the *Classic of Difficulties* has also introduced the concept of "regulating qi" (tido qi) with acupuncture. This is an often under-utilized treatment approach in the modern clinic. The techniques translated in English as tonifying and draining are actually describing a fairly subtle alteration of movement which involves changing the qi dynamic. By altering the movement of qi in the channels, a chain reaction is initiated which alters the qi dynamic and eventually leads to noticeable physiological change.[3]

Thus, while Chapter 78 introduces the concept that one might tonify or drain in general, Chapter 72 points out that acupuncture can also regulate. Basically, Chapter 72 is elaborating on the concepts presented in Chapter 78 to include the actual results of tonifying or draining channel flow. When one changes the flow, the net effect might be called "regulation": This is especially

---

3   Wang, J. & Robertson, J. (2008) *Applied Channel Theory in Chinese Medicine: Wang Ju-Yi's Lectures on Channel Therapeutics.* Seattle, WA: Eastland Press.

important to keep in mind when thinking about how acupuncture affects physiology.[4]

The Back Transporting points affect the organs directly and are therefore used in Interior diseases of the Yin or Yang organs. This is a very important aspect of the clinical effect of these points. They act in quite a different way to all the other points. When treating the Internal Organs, other points work by stimulating the Qi of the channel, which then flows along the channel like a wave, eventually reaching the Internal Organs. In my experience, when we needle the Back Transporting points, Qi goes *directly* to the relevant organ, not through the intermediary of its channel.[5]

Giovanni Maciocia says that the stimulation of points creates a wave of Qi from the point through the channel and to the organ if the goal is to treat the organ. The wave he describes is movement inside the channel and that movement has a direction—to an area or away from an area—which is directed by a reinforcing or reducing needling technique. The needling technique guides treatments. It is the practitioner's skill in creating the "wave" that leads to clinical effectiveness, and is essential in treatment.

Acupoint is a neutral receiver of stimulation; it has no tonifying or sedating characteristic of its own: it responds to the technique applied to it. If one uses the reinforcing technique it will be reinforced and if one uses a sedating technique on an acupoint it will be reduced.[6]

That is a clear explanation that the practitioner's needling method is the key in stimulating a point and channel to achieve the clinical objective—reinforcing or reducing. Points have no specific function of their own, they only respond to stimulation.

4 Ibid.
5 Maciocia, G. (2005) *The Foundations of Chinese Medicine: A Comprehensive Text for Acupuncturists and Herbalists.* Oxford: Churchill Livingstone.
6 Wang, Z. & Wang, J. (2007) *Ling Shu Acupuncture.* Irvine, CA: Ling Shu Press.

Nei dan

Nei dan is Chinese internal meditation. There are many traditions with shared and differing methods. One common method is to circulate Qi throughout the body; some of the practices include circulating Qi through the main channels, the Eight Extraordinary Channels and the internal organs. A way qi gong practitioners circulate Qi throughout the body is with their yi (intention); this is focusing attention at areas of the body. There is a famous saying: *where the mind/attention/yi goes, Qi will follow*. The locations of attention can vary; common practices follow a channel flow from beginning to end. By moving one's attention through a channel, Qi follows it. With practice, Qi is felt and the sensation can range from slight to strong. The sensation of Qi becomes undeniable.

Tai chi chuan is one of the most effective ways to circulate Qi throughout the body to feel its movement. Practicing qi gong, nei dan and tai chi chuan for many years led me to the insight that this process should be followed in the practice of acupuncture. This experience taught me that we are not in the hope business in clinical practice. By that I mean that we do not just hope our treatments move to the targeted area. Instead, it is most effective to take an active role in sending the influence of a treatment to the targeted areas in a similar way a herbalist includes guiding herbs in a formula. For example, if the goal is to reinforce the Spleen and the point combination is Spleen 3 and Spleen 9, the stream/source and sea points, the "hope" is that by reinforcing those two points there will be an increase of Qi flow to the Spleen to reinforce it and restore it to its normal function. Treating two points creates more movement than one point.

Being able to feel the Qi sensation from practicing nei dan and tai chi chuan for decades guided me to add one more point to the two-point combination of Spleen 3 and Spleen 9—the destination point.

For more information on nei dan, see my book *Taoist Nei Dan Inner Meditation: An Accessible Guide*.

Destination treatments

Nei Jing confirms the importance of including the destination in treatments. Chapter 26 of *Su Wen*, "The Relation between the Weather Change and the Eight Main Solar Terms and the Purging and Invigorating by Acupuncture," presents the importance of including destination in treatments. One translation is as follows:

> In employing tonification techniques one must grasp the state of roundness. What is meant by roundness? Round refers to flow, the flow of qi. This refers to guiding the qi to the place of deficit.[7]

The following is another translation of Chapter 26 of *Su Wen*:

> In invigorating therapy, "dredging" means to activate the energy, and activating means to induct the energy to the location of focus.[8]

Reinforcing

Adding the destination point directs the treatment exactly to the targeted area. For example, including Liver 13, the Spleen front mu point, to Spleen 3 and Spleen 9 directs Qi right into the Spleen. Adding the destination point removes the "hope" part of the treatment. Inserting needles in the order of Spleen 3, Spleen 9, and then Liver 13 is a clear message to the body that the treatment is the Spleen channel and the Spleen organ. The order of needle insertion stimulates and guides Qi directly to the organ. The three points work together to stimulate one channel to guide Qi to the destination—the Spleen. Three points and three stimulations cause circulation, which moves Qi to the destination; this is a local-distal points combination, and it is in every standard acupuncture book used in acupuncture schools. Sometimes, one

---

7   Ni, M. (1995) *The Yellow Emperor's Classic of Medicine: A New Translation of Neijing Suwen with Commentary*. Boston, MA: Shambhala.
8   Wu, N. & Wu, A. (2002) *Yellow Emperor's Canon of Internal Medicine*. Beijing: China Science Technology Press.

point can be effective, while at other times two, three or more are necessary; that can be determined in the treatment as the practitioner responds to the patient.

Reducing

When there is a reducing treatment plan, begin the treatment at the location to be reduced and then needle away from it. For example, if there is Liver fire (or any Liver excess), insert the first needle at Liver 14, the front mu of the Liver, reduce it and then select other points on the channel. There can be variations—one combination can be Liver 14, Liver 8, Liver 3 (or Liver 2). Another combination can be Liver 14 and Liver 2. The destination of a reducing treatment is outward, away, and can be downward. Always move away from the problem location for imbalances that require a reducing method.

Whether the treatment plan is to reinforce or reduce, the objective is creating a force (movement, circulation, vibration, stimulation, intensity) to cause the body/channel/organ or area to move either inward to an area or outward and away. The number of areas to treat, the needle sequence direction and the strength of stimulation all combine to create the therapeutic effect.

Three main parts to direction-based treatments

1. The first part of a direction-based treatment is identifying the location of the condition—that area is the center (target) of the treatment plan.

2. The second part of the treatment plan is determining if the condition is excess or deficient. The condition determines the directionality of the treatment and the needle sequence.

Deficient conditions require reinforcing and the movement is toward an area. When there is a reinforcing treatment, the destination is generally an internal organ; the mu or shu point is generally the destination acupuncture point in that situation. Mu and shu points are local to the internal organs and directly influence them more than any other acupuncture points. The movement for a reinforcing treatment is toward the destination. For example, Lung 1 is the destination point when reinforcing the Lung, while Ren 12 is the destination point when reinforcing the Stomach. A reinforcing treatment for the Stomach would be to treat Stomach 36, Stomach 30 and then Ren 12 (the mu point), in that order.

Excess conditions require a reducing technique; the movement created is away and/or outward from where the excess is located. A reducing treatment begins at the location of the excess or close to it, and the treatment movement is away, meaning the body is stimulated to move the excess. For example, you might treat Stomach 21 and then Stomach 44 for Stomach heat, or Lung 5 and then Lung 11 for heat in the Lung. It is more effective to begin the treatment at the location of the excess; for the lung, this would mean treating Lung 1 and then Lung 5 and Lung 11. The order is the key to this treatment approach; it activates the strongest directional circulation within the channel.

The reinforcing needling sequence begins distal to the local area of the condition and moves to the destination. For example, to reinforce the Liver, the needling sequence is Liver 3, Liver 8 and then Liver 14.

The reducing needling sequence begins local to the condition and moves away to the distal area of treatment. For example, treat Stomach 21 and then Stomach 44 when treating Stomach fire (Stomach heat or any excess in the

Stomach; it is not pathogen or pattern limited and it reduces the channel/organ).

3. The third part of a direction-based treatment is to apply the needling technique that matches the condition and the treatment plan.

A reinforcing technique creates a movement in the channels that flows to a destination. Reinforcing two or more areas creates a synergy greater than one area of treatment. A reducing technique creates a movement outward, away and mostly downward from the location of the excess. Reducing two or more areas creates a synergy greater than one area of treatment. Stimulating two or more acupuncture points requires less needling force than trying to get one acupuncture point to match the more gentle stimulation of multiple acupuncture points. Needling multiple acupuncture points allows for thinner needles to achieve the treatment goal. It can be a gentler treatment.

Whether one, two, three or more points on a channel are treated, they are viewed as one group working together as a unified action creating clinically effective movement. They should not be viewed from the individual functions listed in texts.

In the same way that Qi flows where the mind/attention moves when practicing tai chi chuan, qi gong and nei dan, *Qi flows where the needles go*. Sequence the needles and the treatment to create the optimal flow of Qi.

CHAPTER 4

Reinforcing and Reducing Channels

Chinese-Asian medicine includes a variety of models and theories that practitioners use to make a diagnosis and develop a treatment plan. Theories are placed above the channel system and the practitioner often thinks the activity of the "theory" is what occurs in the channels. The *Nan Ching* writers assigned five phases to the five transporting points and created the basis for a five-phases acupuncture point treatment. In this approach, the five-phases points are selected based on their phase (five element) relationship to the channel, not the ability of the acupuncture point to stimulate the body when a needling technique is applied. For example, Heart 7 is the earth point on the fire heart channel and it is the five-phases child (reducing/sedating) point—from a five-phases viewpoint, Heart 7 reduces the Heart Fire Channel. The "theory activity" is the five-phases relationship of earth reducing fire; therefore, the channel is reduced. A reducing technique must be applied. From a channel perspective, not a five-phases perspective, applying a reducing technique on Heart 7 will create an outward and away movement in the channel and body. Additionally, including Heart 3 with Heart 7 in that order combines two points, creating a needle sequence, and a needle technique to reduce. In my experience, that will be more effective than treating one point to reduce a channel or organ.

Five-phases theory directs selecting Heart 7, the earth point on a fire channel, to reduce the Heart channel. A classical channel-based approach guides one to apply either a reducing or reinforcing needling technique to any acupuncture point. The choice of why to select an acupuncture point to treat is different between five-phases theory and a channel-needling technique-based approach. In basic five-phases theory, only the child is selected to reduce a channel. In a channel-needling technique-based approach any acupuncture point can be selected and treated with the appropriate needling technique. The needling technique determines the acupuncture activity of reinforcing or reducing.

Often the original structure and function of the channels is removed from the practitioner's understanding of how acupuncture works. This chapter will explain how understanding the original function (based on classical theory) of the channels can become the basis of creating acupuncture treatments.

Common teaching

Learning the functions of each individual acupuncture point is the standard presentation in schools. It is common for the student to think that each point can treat all the conditions and syndromes that are listed for each acupuncture point. This approach prevents the practitioner from understanding the relationship between channels and acupuncture points and removes the reality of the synergy (multiple areas of stimulation working together to achieve the same objective) that is created by treating multiple points on a channel.

In the study of acupuncture, students learn the pathways of the channels. The internal pathways flow deep within the body and their trajectories flow to where the acupuncture points exist at the more superficial layers. Each of the twelve main channels' trajectories links to its own organ and its Yin-Yang paired organ. The link between a channel and an internal organ is the reason a distal treatment for treating organs can be effective. *That link is just a link—it is not a blood link, a body fluid link, an essence link, a Yin link or Yang link; it is a channel link that can be influenced to reduce or reinforce.*

No Yin, No Yang—only Qi

Yin-Yang is not Qi. Qi is often named by its location and function. Yuan qi originates in the Kidneys, gu qi in the Stomach/Spleen, and zong qi in the chest. Ying qi and wei qi are derived from zong qi. Wei qi flows to the superficial layers, and Ying qi flows in the acupuncture channels (*Ling Shu*, Chapter 16, "Nourishing Qi"). In this model, Qi is not defined as Yin qi or Yang qi. In the acupuncture channels, there is no Yin qi or Yang qi; there is only Qi (bioelectricity). When there is a diagnosis of Kidney Yang qi deficiency, there is no individual acupuncture point or set of acupuncture points that can definitively be characterized as more Yang than Yin or more Yin than Yang. The Yin-Yang model is used to identify imbalances. Acupuncture is a way to influence a channel within the body to regain balance. The ability of acupuncture to create therapeutic movement to restore the underlying condition (excess or deficiency) and therefore balance either a Yin or Yang imbalance is the unique healing quality of acupuncture.

Table 4.1 shows the main signs and symptoms from imbalances of the Liver. When there is a deficiency of the Liver, the treatment plan is to reinforce the Liver. Creating movement (standard acupuncture language is circulating Qi) into the Liver will bring it into balance, correcting the imbalance. There is no other treatment than filling the Liver with Qi. Stimulating the Liver channel to move Qi until the therapeutic effect occurs is the objective of treatment. The primary goal is to fill the Liver (or any organ) until it functions in a balanced way, which means being able to perform its normal functions. There is no lock and key phenomenon related to one acupuncture point treating specific signs, symptoms, pathogens and patterns. The zangfu systemization of

CLINICAL POINT SELECTION

acupuncture point functions is a rigid oversimplification that leads to a misunderstanding of how acupuncture functions and how to create acupuncture treatments.

When there is Liver excess, the treatment plan is to reduce. This is the treatment plan for any of the numerous types of excess. Note that in Table 4.1 the treatment in the last column is the same for all the different patterns and signs and symptoms. The goal in a reducing treatment plan is to stimulate the channel enough to clear and move the excess. Acupuncture reducing techniques cannot distinguish what is reduced, so all of the excesses are reduced.

Table 4.1. Summary of Liver patterns and symptoms

Condition	Pattern	Treatment
Liver excess patterns	Liver qi stagnation, Liver blood stagnation, Liver fire, Liver wind, Liver Yang rising, dampness or heat in the Liver, cold in the Liver	Reduce
Liver excess signs and symptoms	Hypochondriac pain, sighing, hiccuping, belching, nausea, vomiting, abdominal distention, irregular periods, distention of the breasts before the period, premenstrual syndrome, melancholy, moodiness, anger, irritability, resentment, dizziness, red face and eyes, bitter taste, tremor, numbness, vomiting, headache, constipation	Reduce
Liver deficiency	Liver blood deficiency, Liver Yin deficiency	Reinforce
Liver deficiency signs and symptoms	Dizziness, numbness of the limbs, muscle spasms, amenorrhea, floaters, dry eyes, dry skin, headache, tinnitus, insomnia, blurred vision, muscular weakness, brittle nails, temporal headaches, irritability, dream-disturbed sleep, pale lips, sallow complexion, tic or tremor of the hands and feet	Reinforce

Liver 3 is often needled to treat Liver blood deficiency; it is a source point and it strongly influences the channel and organ. I would emphasize that it is selected to reinforce the Liver (Liver blood in this case) because it strongly stimulates the channel and the Qi in

50

REINFORCING AND REDUCING CHANNELS

it, not because it has a unique influence on Liver blood. An acupuncture treatment is not treating Liver blood, it is strengthening the Liver so that it works properly and generates the substances it produces. A five-phases (five element) practitioner may treat Liver 8, the sea, water and five-phases parent-reinforcing point to treat Liver blood deficiency, Liver Yin deficiency, Liver qi stagnation or damp heat in the Liver. The acupuncture treatment does not treat those substances, it treats the channel/organ that creates them. With a reinforcing needling technique, it will stimulate movement to the Liver—both Liver 3 and Liver 8 treat Liver Yin and Liver blood deficiency, as well as Liver qi and Liver blood stagnation. They treat those conditions and potentially any condition of the Liver because they can be needled to stimulate the channel/organ.

Confirm this reality by reviewing a few standard texts on acupuncture point functions. Looking beneath the zangfu language, those two points do not treat those vital substances (Liver blood, Liver Yin), they treat the Liver channel and organ to restore the organ's ability to generate those vital substances. The treatment goal is to restore the organ to function normally (as close as possible) so it will then function properly. This is true for all the organs. Understanding that mechanism is essential in creating channel-needling, technique-based acupuncture treatments.

The special category acupuncture points (source, transporting, mu, shu, etc.) have a strong effect on the channels/organs as they are not limited to the specific functions listed in a point category. Points in those categories can treat any excess or deficiency condition; they strongly stimulate the movement in the channels to reinforce or reduce the channel/organ. Different models lead the practitioner to view and use an acupuncture point in a specific way, which is a narrow way. For example, in the five-phases Heart 7, Shen Men is an earth point and the five-phases child and sedation acupuncture point, and it is used to reduce an excess. It would reduce any excess as the five-phases model is not zangfu organ pattern based. Heart 7 is also the source point; in channel-based acupuncture it is the needling technique that determines if Heart

7 reinforces or reduces—that reality is true regardless of the theory used to select and treat acupuncture points.

Embryonic stem cells and Qi

Embryonic stem cells have unlimited healing potential because they are the building blocks of the human body. They are unspecialized and can develop into specific cells; they offer the possibility to treat any organ, gland or area of the human body. Qi is similar. At the basis of all is Qi: all the other vital substances are but manifestations of Qi. Qi gong, tai chi chuan and qi gong healing practitioners influence health by circulating, gathering, directing and storing Qi to specific areas of the body. There is no definitive difference in the quality of the Qi. If a person is Qi deficient, Qi is the solution. And it is the solution for each organ, gland and area of the body. The channels are the medium to distribute Qi, and Qi can restore an organ to balance. The balance will show with the diagnostic models that include visual inspection, questioning and pulse and tongue diagnosis. Yin-Yang is a tool for analysis; it is not the substance to treat imbalances. Qi is the substance for healing. The practitioner influences an acupuncture channel and the Qi in it. The result is reflected with diagnostic models.

Only Qi in the channels

It is often taught that Kidney 3 treats Kidney Yin and Kidney 7 treats Kidney Yang; however, this is a misleading categorization of acupuncture point functions. If one looks at any major acupuncture text, it will say that one point can treat many conditions—for example, Kidney 3 can treat Kidney Yin deficiency, Kidney Yang deficiency, Kidney qi deficiency and Kidney essence deficiency. How can it do all that? Are all those qualities inside the area of Kidney 3? Is there earth inside Kidney 3 because it is an earth point and is there metal inside Kidney 7 because it is a metal point? Yin-Yang and five phases are models that identify the condition of an organ system (and areas of the body). The key is that there is only Qi in the channels and when Qi is directed to an organ or area to reinforce it, the Qi energizes and restores it to a balanced state, which can be identified by standard diagnostic tools of Chinese medicine—there are levels of restoration due to the nature of the condition and the patient. This reality is reflected in the following statement: "All the various types of qi are one qi merely manifesting in different forms."[1] That nature of Qi allows it to benefit any imbalance and area of the body. This is the unique nature of Qi and acupuncture that makes it different from herbal medicine.

In *Foundations of Chinese Medicine*, Giovanni Maciocia presents acupuncture point combinations for the main patterns and syndromes for the internal organs. Evaluating the point combinations reveals that the same points treat multiple internal organ patterns. For example, Spleen 3 and 6 treat Spleen qi deficiency, Spleen Yang deficiency, Spleen blood deficiency and Spleen qi sinking. This type of pattern and point combination occurs for all the channels. Organizing acupuncture point functions by their channel instead of function reveals that numerous points on a channel treat the same condition—they treat the same channel and organ and their imbalances. It is most important to identify the acupuncture points and areas that create the strongest movement, which is a reinforcing or reducing movement, to create effective treatments. Understanding this dynamic is necessary to shift to a channel-based style of clinical point selection.

Zangfu pattern differentiation includes identifying the imbalanced channel/organ and the type of pathogen or vital substance that is in excess or deficiency, and then treating them. The zangfu model is suitable for herbal medicine. It is not suitable for acupuncture, meaning it's not highly effective for acupuncture treatments. In acupuncture, the channels are influenced with a

---

1   Maciocia, G. (2005) *The Foundations of Chinese Medicine: A Comprehensive Text for Acupuncturists and Herbalists*. Oxford: Churchill Livingstone.

needling technique, either reinforcing or reducing. Whatever is in the channel is reduced (sedated, cleared, moved, etc.), there is no pathogen differential, meaning no one point can definitively treat one pathogen over another. The entire channel is influenced and whatever is in the channel is reduced. The same occurs when the reinforcing technique is applied. Reinforcing stimulates the channel to move the channel and the bio-electricity (Qi) to an organ and area to restore it, increasing its ability to produced its vital substances. The treatment plan is to restore the organ function, not reinforce a particular substance. The organ will generate what has not been generated. There are no acupuncture points that definitively restore a particular substance. Understanding this reality allows the practitioner to have the widest range of acupuncture point selection strategies. All traditions that include treating the imbalanced channels directly are included in this approach. The goal is to stimulate the channel to accomplish the treatment plan; combining acupuncture points to stimulate the channel is the guiding principle in this channel-based acupuncture points selection system.

Looking beneath the models laid on top of the channels reveals that there is only bio-electricity (Qi) in the channels, and Qi has the capacity to influence any organ or area of the body—that influence (change) will be reflected in the Yin-Yang, five-phases and zangfu models of diagnosis. The treatment strategy is to stimulate the channel to create a reaction/movement/circulation—either reinforcing or reducing through the channel system and body to obtain the desired effect. For example, an organ can be the targeted location, the channel is the transportation system and the acupuncture points (or areas along the channel) are the locations for stimulating the channel. Channels, acupuncture points, destination and Qi comprise one inseparable system. It is the ability of the practitioner to stimulate this system that significantly contributes to clinical effectiveness. Guided by the understanding that there is no Yin and Yang qi but only Qi in the practice of acupuncture, the practitioner expands the possibilities for creating acupuncture treatments.

CHAPTER 5

The Conduit Vessels: The Main Channels

Chapter 10 of the *Ling Shu*, "The Conduit Vessels," presents the twelve main channels that are connected to the internal organs, which are the most common channels treated in TCM. In that chapter, there are no acupuncture points listed on the main channels; instead, only the channel pathways are presented. Signs, symptoms and conditions are listed for imbalances of each channel, as well as the pulse method (Renying-Cunkou) that measures them. Chapter 9 of the *Ling Shu*, "End and Beginning," presents the Renying-Cunkou pulse method and combined with Chapter 10, presents a system for diagnosis, treatment and measurement. One of the most important aspects of this system is to treat imbalanced channels directly.

Chapter 59 in *Su Wen*, titled "Pathways of the Channels," describes how the Qi of the acupuncture channels forms the acupuncture points in a way that indicates it is the entire channel that should be the primary emphasis of treatment, while the formal acupuncture points are just one way to stimulate the channel to treat a condition.

> The acupoints issued from the Foot Taiyin channel's energy are seventy-three. The acupoints issued from the Foot Shaoyang channel's energy are sixty-two. The acupoints issued from the Foot Yangming channel are sixty-eight.[1]

---

1 Wang, Z. & Wang, J. (2007) *Ling Shu Acupuncture*. Irvine, CA: Ling Shu Press.

> The acupuncture points are emanated and formed by the Qi/Blood of the Foot-Taiyang Meridian are seventy-eight points bilaterally.[2]

The following is commentary from *Ling Shu Acupuncture*:

> The significance of the above statement made the function and the indication of the acupoint concrete. The indications of an acupoint are the symptoms that are associated with the dysfunctions of the pertaining meridian. In other words, the functions and indications of each acupoint are related to its pertaining meridian only.
>
> In *Ling Shu* chapter 10 it was stated that the symptoms are due to the dysfunction of each meridian. Those symptoms are the indications for all the acupoints of the Lung Meridian.[3]

All the quotes explain that the meridians form the acupuncture points, and the function of the points is based on the function of the meridians. This relationship explains why all points on a meridian have the potential to treat the imbalances of a meridian. It is evident after studying *Nei Jing* and subsequent texts that how acupuncture works is that it creates movement within the channels, and the primary goal in treatment is to strategically stimulate the channels. *Nei Jing*'s method to stimulate the channels is applying a reinforcing or reducing technique. Understanding this mechanism allows greater flexibility in selecting areas for treatment and transcends a rigid one-point-treats-all approach.

Where acupuncture occurs

In a similar way that a neurosurgeon understands and works with the innervation and vascular systems, the acupuncturist should know and work with the entire channel system. It is not a mistake that the channel system is presented in every curriculum at

---

2   Ibid.
3   Ibid.

Chinese medical schools, and this usually happens first, before the acupuncture points are presented. The acupuncture channel structure is where Qi and blood flow. It is where pathogenic factors can lodge, and it is where the practitioner can influence the body and the flow of Qi and blood to clear blockages and reinforce organs. The ability of the practitioner to effectively apply acupuncture techniques creates the acupuncture activity in the channels and generates the desired therapeutic effect. The therapeutic effect is alluded to in *Nei Jing* but not in clear, focused explanations. Treating channels via acupuncture points and areas on the imbalanced channel(s) is the most important principle in creating acupuncture treatments. The acupuncture treatment approaches in this book will include how to influence a channel by strategically creating movement within the channels to achieve the treatment goal.

CHAPTER 6

Channel Selection

Acupuncture is primarily a location-based treatment method—identify the location of the condition and treat it with a variation of local and distal points and areas with channels that flow to the location. The *Ling Shu* presents multiple acupuncture treatment approaches that include treating individual acupuncture points and areas along the channels. The common method practiced is treating individual acupuncture points and combining them in a hodgepodge way. I propose that strategically selecting channels first and then selecting combinations of points and areas for treatment is essential for clinical efficacy. The following *Ling Shu* quotes guide the practitioner to treat a specific channel, not a particular acupuncture point. Chapter 24 of *Ling Shu*, "The Receding [Qi] Diseases," states:

> Low back pain. When the pain is accompanied by cold moving upward, one chooses the foot major Yang [conduits for piercing the needle]... If a headache results from receding [Qi is accompanied by] dizziness and a feeling of heaviness and pin in the head. The hand minor Yin [conduit] is chosen first. After that one chooses the foot minor Yin [conduit for piercing the needle]... Toothache. If it is not accompanied by an aversion to cool beverages. One chooses the foot Yang brilliance [conduit for piercing the needle].[1]

In addition, Chapter 22 of the *Ling Shu*, "Peak Illness and Madness,"

---

[1] Unschuld, P. (2016) *Huang Di Nei Jing Ling Shu: The Ancient Classic on Needle Therapy*. University of California Press.

explains, "When there is insanity and speech, it is accompanied by fright. Treat the Arm Bright Yang, Arm Major Yang and Arm Major Yin."[2]

Needling sequence

The quotes above reveal that the practitioner should select channels first, and then determine the effective points and areas for treatment. The ipsilateral treatment sequencing is presented in this book. It is generally more effective to needle up or down one side of a channel to create a stronger influence than to treat the right side and then the left side and back and forth, which diminishes the momentum (movement, circulation, therapeutic force) in a channel. The ipsilateral sequence is essential in creating an effective therapeutic effect within a channel.

Channel combinations

It is often necessary to strategically select supporting channels in treatment. The *Ling Shu* clearly presents treating Yin-Yang paired channels in treatment; that is the first supporting channel to consider in an acupuncture plan. *Yin-Yang paired channels intersect with their own and their paired organ; that is why they can treat (influence) each other, and I would argue that is why they are Yin-Yang paired channels.* My preference for additional supporting channels is for ones that interact with the imbalanced channel; the six-channel pair is a common choice as the second supporting channel, especially when combining hand and foot channels in treatment. Any channel that intersects (internal pathway intersections) with the imbalanced channel is an option too. The channels can be combined into two-, three- and four-channel

---

2 Ibid.

treatments. The following section presents these approaches to channel selection.

Two-channel combination: Yin-Yang paired channels

Chapter 9 of the *Ling Shu*, "From Beginning to End," presents treating Yin-Yang paired channels in each treatment. The method is based on the Renying-Cunkou pulse diagnostic and treatment method, which identifies the imbalanced channel. Yin-Yang paired channels are always treated together in this approach—this is a two-channel treatment plan. The two channels intersect with each other via the internal pathways; therefore, they influence each other due to their intersection. As the two channels are stimulated, they work together to accomplish the therapeutic effect. Two channels create a stronger influence than one channel. For example, if there is Liver qi stagnation, treat Liver 8 and Liver 3, and then treat Gallbladder 34 and Gallbladder 41. This acupuncture point combination is composed of the sea and stream points on the Yin-Yang paired channels, which create a stronger influence than treating one channel. The practitioner can apply the ipsilateral, alternating or completion sequence.

In addition to Chapter 9 of the *Ling Shu*, there are other chapters that recommend using Yin-Yang pairs in treatment. For instance, Chapter 28 of the *Ling Shu*, "Questions on the Oral Teachings," states, "When the Yin qi is exhausted, and the Yang qi is full, it causes one to wake from sleep. Disperse leg minor Yin and tonify leg major Yang."[3] Chapter 22 of the *Ling Shu*, "Peak Illness and Madness," explains, "When there is insanity and speech, it is accompanied by fright. Treat the Arm Bright Yang, Arm Major Yang and Arm Major Yin."[4]

---

3   Wu, J. (2002) *Ling Shu or The Spiritual Pivot*. Hawaii: University of Hawaii Press.
4   Unschuld, P. (2016) *Huang Di Nei Jing Ling Shu: The Ancient Classic on Needle Therapy*. University of California Press.

Three-channel combination: Yin-Yang paired channels and one six-channel pair

Treating Yin-Yang paired channels involves combining two channels to work together to treat the imbalanced channel. Adding the six-channel pair of the imbalanced channel to the Yin-Yang pairs involves three channels working together to treat the imbalanced channel. For example, if the Spleen is deficient, adding the Stomach and the Lung channels is adding the Yin-Yang and Taiyin pair of the Spleen to the treatment. This channel combination offers additional support to the treatment. The addition of the six-channel pair is used when the Yin-Yang pair alone is not effective.

> **EXAMPLE**
>
> A patient is diagnosed with Spleen qi deficiency. The treatment is to reinforce Spleen 3 and Spleen 9, then treat Stomach 43 and 36, and finish by treating Lung 9 and 5. The Spleen and Stomach are Yin-Yang paired channels, and the Lung is the Taiyin pair of the Spleen. Treat the Lung channel, the Taiyin-paired channel of the Spleen (foot Taiyin), last.

Four-channel combination: Yin-Yang and six-channel pairs

Combining Yin-Yang and six-channel paired channels involves using four channels to treat the imbalanced channel—this brings together four influences (forces) working as one. For example, when the Liver is in excess, treating the Liver, Gallbladder, Pericardium and San Jiao means to use the four-channel circuit where Yin-Yang pairs and their six-channel pairs are combined to create a strong therapeutic effect.

The four-channel combination is based on the Ying qi circuit presented in Chapter 16 of the *Ling Shu*, "The Nourishing Qi" (this cycle is commonly known as the daily or meridian clock): Lung, Large Intestine, Stomach and Spleen; Heart, Small Intestine, Bladder and Kidney; and Pericardium, San Jiao, Gallbladder and Liver. This sequence is the common format in which the channels are presented in acupuncture texts. The meridian clock order of the channels follows Yin-Yang, six-channel and internal-pathway interactions. The Yin-Yang and six-channel combinations link to each other in a circuit and influence each other; this combination is a four-channel treatment. For instance, when the Liver is excess, treat the Liver, Gallbladder, Pericardium and San Jiao channels to create a stronger therapeutic (movement, circulation) effect than treating one, two or three of the channels.

> **EXAMPLE**
>
> Treating Liver 3, Gallbladder 41, Pericardium 7 and San Jiao 3 is a Yin-Yang/six-channel paired treatment. If one point on each channel is not effective, add another layer of the pattern: Liver 8, Gallbladder 34, Pericardium 3 and San Jiao 10. The first layer of points contains the stream points and the second layer contains the sea points; it is a stream-and-sea-point combination.

A channel-based approach to creating acupuncture treatments is a flexible approach to acupuncture point selection. The practitioner can select a wide range of acupuncture points and areas to treat. Select from a wide range of acupuncture point categories for treatment, including five transporting, source, five-phases points, mu and shu points and areas based on palpation. Apply this guidance in practice and not a rigid acupuncture points combination.

Internal-pathway connection treatments

The internal-pathway approach to acupuncture point selection was inspired by my nei dan practice and knowledge of internal pathways and meeting points. The internal-pathway connection method utilizes specific acupuncture channel circuits within the body. A nei dan practice includes moving one's attention (focus/yi) throughout the body to result in a feeling and sensation of Qi in the natural pathways in the body. The practice of acupuncture can work in that way too—for example, treating Lung qi deficiency using pathway circuits that flow to the Lung. The Lungs originate in the Middle Jiao, the Stomach. By tonifying the Stomach, the Lung will benefit; that is the parent nourishing the child in the five phases. Treating Stomach 36 and then Ren 12 brings more Qi into the stomach. Continue the treatment by adding Ren 17 and then Lung 1 to increase the natural flow of Qi through the existing channel system. The Ren channel flows from Ren 12 to Ren 17—the influential point of Qi—and then flows to the Lung. Treating Ren 17 and then Lung 1 enhances the normal flow through the channels to reinforce the Lung. It is important to add the destination point, Lung 1, to direct Qi to the Lung. Both the Spleen and the Stomach channels flow to the Stomach/Ren 12. Creating treatments that increase the flow of Qi to the Stomach (or any organ) is also guiding the treatment to the Lung via the normal pathways of the channels.

It is the sequence of acupuncture points and areas of treatment that guides the treatment to specific areas. Adding Lung 1, the destination point, takes the hope out of the treatment and sends the treatment more effectively to the targeted location. If the condition is very deficient, combine the Spleen and the Stomach channels to support the Lungs. An example of this internal pathway approach is treating Stomach 43 and then Stomach 36, and then treating Spleen 3 and then Spleen 9. In this treatment, the Stomach and Spleen channels are reinforced to guide Qi to Ren 12, where it will flow into the Lungs. Ideally, the Stomach and Spleen channels and Ren 12 are treated for 15–20 minutes before Ren 17 and Lung 1 are treated. In my experience, this type of treatment is significantly more effective than treating the Lung channel alone or with its Yin-Yang paired channel, the Large Intestine channel.

After the Yin-Yang paired channel, I prefer to use internal pathway connections as supporting channels.

Treatment types

Channel-based treatments have a channel and acupuncture point sequence which when applied can increase clinical effectiveness. The sequence begins with the primary treatment, which includes treating the imbalanced channel(s) and then the Yin-Yang paired channel. The secondary and supporting treatments are related channels, which can be the six-channel paired channel and internal pathway connections. The third aspect of a treatment can include systemic points, which may treat the body systemically, not just the channel/organ. For instance, He Gu, Large Intestine 4 treats pain anywhere in the body. The fourth aspect of a treatment is selecting channels and points throughout the body that may treat the condition, but may not have any channel or organ relationship. Points in that category are often called *empirical points*.

Identifying channel(s) that require treatment is the first step in developing an acupuncture treatment plan; including channels that have the strongest relationship to the imbalanced channel(s) is the most direct and clinically effective approach to selecting channel combinations.

Targeting treatment

Primary aspect of a treatment: The shortest distance between two points is a straight line. A straight line is treating the imbalance channel that flows directly to the area to be treated. When that approach is implemented, it is the *primary treatment*, it is a direct channel treatment to the targeted area.

Secondary aspect of a treatment: The secondary aspect of a treatment is adding a supporting channel to treat the primary channel being treated. Classically, adding the Yin-Yang paired channel of the primary treatment is the second most direct channel for treatment as it flows to the organ of the primary channel and is another channel that flows to the targeted organ.

Tertiary aspect of a treatment include treating channels that have a connection to the targeted area, for example a channel with an internal pathway that flows to the targeted area.

Quaternary aspect of a treatment can be channels (phases/elements) that have a relationship to the targeted area, for example the Lungs are the metal phase, it is the parent of water and the Kidneys. In five-phases theory, the parent can nourish or reinforce the child, and Lungs can reinforce the Kidneys based on the five-phases theory, not a channel connection.

I created the name of the treatments above, but you can use any language you prefer to describe the type of treatment. The important aspect of this targeting approach is understanding how the channels selected and treated influence the targeted area based on classical acupuncture channel theory.

CHAPTER 7

Acupuncture Point Categories in the Han Dynasty

The *Nei Jing Su Wen* and *Ling Shu* present main acupuncture point categories practiced in clinics around the world. It's always interesting to discuss what classical acupuncture is with students and practitioners. For the purpose of this book, classical acupuncture is defined by the theories in particular texts, for example the *Nei Jing*, and then applying those theories and clinical applications in clinical practice. Some practitioners apply only the material in the *Nei Jing* in clinical practice—they would be *Nei Jing* classical practitioners. Some practitioners apply material in the *Nan Ching* in clinical practice—they are *Nan Ching* classical practitioners. Many study only modern traditional Chinese medicine, which combines many classical theories and applications with numerous additions during the long history of acupuncture.

It's a worthy pursuit to study the classics and learn the theories and clinical applications in them, allowing the practitioner to know a wide range of approaches to clinical practice. Equally important is having the knowledge to evaluate new theories regarding their origin. The Professional Review Chapter 11 in this book explores how a student or practitioner might do an analysis of a new theory (hypothesis). With professional analysis, a practitioner can make an educated decision on whether to include a treatment approach in their practice.

Wide and narrow acupuncture theories and clinical applications

Acupuncture point categories contain actions and indications which include a wide and narrow understanding about how acupuncture works based on the functions of acupuncture points presented. A wide understanding of acupuncture point actions and indications leads to the widest range of functions of acupuncture points. The wide view contains what I call the original way acupuncture works—it's similar to looking under the hood of an automobile to see the inner workings of the engine.

Five phases, zangfu and six stages are common models of Chinese medicine that categorize (filter) information in a narrow view based on its unique theory, because each model generally excludes other views. Narrow theories have pros and cons, and knowing that allows the practitioner to change theories when a different approach could lead to increased clinical efficacy. The *Nei Jing* and *Nan Ching* offer both wide and narrow theories with clinical applications about acupuncture point categories and acupuncture points. Understanding early classical theory and clinical applications is essential in optimizing clinical effectiveness.

Main Han dynasty acupuncture point categories

Source points
Source points (yuan points) are presented in the *Ling Shu*, Chapter 1, "Of Nine Needles and the Twelve Source Points, The Laws of Heaven," and Chapter 2, "The Roots of the Acupuncture Points." *Ling Shu*, Chapter 1 lists the source points for Yin channels; there

are no Yang channel source points in the *Ling Shu*, Chapter 1; they are added in the *Ling Shu*, Chapter 2. In those two chapters and in the *Nan Ching* the broadest use of the source points is presented. It will be other people's views that narrow the usage. From both theory and clinical experience, source points are the most practical and clinically effective acupuncture points to treat any condition of a channel and organ; it is only narrow theories that would limit their functions.

From a translation of the *Ling Shu*, Chapter 1:

> The five long-term depots have six short-term repositories. The six short-term repositories have twelve origin [openings]. The exits of the twelve origin [openings] are in the four key joints. Through the four key joints one controls the therapy of the five long-term depots.
>
> When any of the five long-term depots has an illness, it should be made to leave through the twelve origin [openings]. Each of the twelve origin [openings] has something that exits through it. To clearly know these origin [openings], and to observe their reactions lets one know the type of injury of the five long-term depots.[1]

Ling Shu, translation 2:

> The five viscera have resonances with the six bowels. The six bowels have twelve source points. The twelve source points come out near the four gates. The four gates control the cure of the five viscera.
>
> When the five viscera are diseased, seize the exact points of the twelve sources.
>
> When the five viscera are diseased, there must be a corresponding manifestation in the twelve sources, and particularly with the source point which has the manifestation of the disease.
>
> Understand clearly the source points. Examine their correspondences and know the illnesses of the five viscera.[2]

---

[1] Unschuld, P. (2016) *Huang Di Nei Jing Ling Shu: The Ancient Classic on Needle Therapy*. University of California Press.

[2] Wu, J. (2002) *Ling Shu or The Spiritual Pivot*. Hawaii: University of Hawaii Press.

Table 7.1: The source points

Channel	Yuan source	Name
Lung	Lung 9	Tai Yuan
Large Intestine	Large Intestine 4	He Gu
Stomach	Stomach 42	Chong Yang
Spleen	Spleen 3	Tai Bai
Heart	Heart 7	Shen Men
Small Intestine	Small Intestine 4	Wan Gu
Bladder	Bladder 64	Jing Gu
Kidney	Kidney 3	Tai Xi
Pericardium	Pericardium 7	Da Ling
San Jiao	San Jiao 4	Yang Chi
Gallbladder	Gallbladder 40	Qui Xu
Liver	Liver 3	Tai Chong

In *Nan Ching: The Classic of Difficult Issues*, Difficulty 66 says:

> It is like this. The influences moving below the navel and between the kidneys constitute man's life. They are the source and the basis of the twelve conduits. Hence they are called "original [influences]." The Triple Burner is the special envoy that transmits the original influences. It is responsible for the passage of the three influences through the [body's] five depots and six palaces. "Origin" is an honorable designation for the Triple Burner. Hence [the place] where [its influences] come to a halt is [called] "origin." In case the [body's] five depots and six palaces suffer from an illness, one always selects their respective [conduits'] origin [holes for pricking].[3]

Nei Jing and *Nan Ching* guidance is that the source points can treat any condition of the internal organs, which includes excess and deficiency conditions. *Needling technique* determines whether a

---

[3] Unschuld, P. (1986) *Nan-Ching: The Classic of Difficult Issues*. University of California Press.

treatment is reinforcing or reducing, not a theory of the function of an acupuncture point or channel. Source points treat any condition of the internal organs.

Back shu points

The back shu points are presented in the *Ling Shu*, Chapter 51, "The Back Shu Acupuncture Points." This includes the five Yin organ back shu points and Ge Shu, Bladder 17, the back shu of the diaphragm. There are six back shu points listed in the *Ling Shu*. The other back shu points begin to appear in literature with *The Pulse Classic (Jing Ming)* and then in *The Systematic Classic of Acupuncture (Jia Yi Jing)*. Below are examples of the *Ling Shu* presentation of the back shu points.

Ling Shu, Chapter 51, "The Back Shu Acupuncture Points":

> Qi Bo said, In the middle of the back are the great shu acupuncture points. At the tips of the shuttle bone are the Big Shuttle points.
>
> The lung shu points are located at the gaps of the third vertebra.
>
> The diaphragm shu points are located at the gaps of the seventh vertebra.
>
> The kidney shu points are located at the gaps of fourteenth vertebra.
>
> Moxibustion can be effective when needling is not effective. When the qi is full, disperse; when hollow, tonify. When using fire to tonify, do not blow on the fire. In a moment it will go out by itself. When using the fire to disperse, quickly blow on the fire to propagate the action of the Artemisia, then extinguish the fire.[4]

The following texts introduced the remaining back shu points: *The Canon of Pulse (Mai Jing)*, *Jia Yi Jing* and the *Prescriptions Worth a Thousand Gold for Emergencies*.

---

4   Wu, J. (2002) *Ling Shu or The Spiritual Pivot*. Hawaii: University of Hawaii Press.

Table 7.2: The 12 back shu points

Channel	Back shu	
Lung	UB 13	Fei Shu
Pericardium	UB 14	Jueyin Xu
Heart	UB 15	Xin Shu
Diaphragm	UB 17	Ge Shu
Liver	UB 18	Gan Shu
Gallbladder	UB 19	Dan Xu
Spleen	UB 20	Pi Shu
Stomach	UB 21	Wei Shu
San Jiao	UB 22	San Jiao Shu
Kidney	UB 23	Shen Xu
Large Intestine	UB 25	Da Chang Xu
Small Intestine	UB 27	Xia Chang Shu
Bladder	UB 28	Pang Gang Shu

The *Ling Shu* does not state that the shu points can be only reinforced or reduced; it is only teachers and practitioners that chose a theory to support a narrow view. The *Ling Shu* presents a reinforcing and reducing moxabustion method. The classical understanding is that a reinforcing or reducing technique can be applied to all acupuncture points, including the shu acupuncture points. A practitioner should research the origins of any theory or tradition that guides a usage different than the original guidance.

Back shu points are local to their corresponding organ; they have the most direct influence on it and are important in the local-distal points acupuncture combination treatment for internal organs. Shu points are destination points. The shu points can be reinforced or reduced. Standard acupuncture books include combining shu points with other points, for example source points, to treat the internal organs. The needling technique determines if the treatment is reinforcing or reducing.

The shu points are used as a diagnostic method to determine

imbalances of the internal organs. These points reflect the condition of the organ, they correspond to them. If there is heat in the organ it can appear or show at the points; it can feel hot or look red.

Front mu points

Front mu points are not listed in the *Ling Shu* and *Su Wen*. There is a mention of mu points in Chapter 47 of the *Su Wen*:

> Huang Di asked, What is the cause of a bitter taste in the mouth that is relieved after treating the gallbladder point yanglingquan? Qi Bo answered, This condition is called dan tan or gallbladder heat. The patient is usually very indecisive and worries a lot. This suppresses the gallbladder function. Thus the bile, instead of being distributed properly, is excreted upward, causing the bitter taste. One must treat using the front mu/alarm point and the back shu/transport point of the gallbladder.[5]

Author note: The *Su Wen* and *Ling Shu* do not list back shu points for Yang organs or any front mu points. The comment regarding them contradicts knowledge in the *Nei Jing*. *The Canon of Pulse* and the *Jia Yi Jing* begin listing the mu points. The mu points are listed as a front mu acupuncture point in the section where the acupuncture points are presented; there is no category of front mu points. There are no indications or actions for the front mu points. Classical clinical application is that the needling technique determines the treatment action; a reinforcing or reducing method can be applied on the mu points, as well as any acupuncture point.

Here is an example of how the *Jia Yi Jing* lists the front mu points:

> Central Venter (*Zhong Wan*, CV 12) is also known as Supreme

---

5   Ni, M. (1995) *The Yellow Emperor's Classic of Medicine: A New Translation of Neijing Suwen with Commentary*. Boston, MA: Shambhala.

CLINICAL POINT SELECTION

Granary (*Tui Cung*). It is the alarm point of the stomach and is located one cun below Upper Venter or at the midpoint between the xiphoid process and the umbilicus.[6]

Front mu points are also called alarm points.

Table 7.3: The front mu points

Channel	Front mu	
Lung	Lung 1	Zhong Fu
Large Intestine	ST 25	Tian Shu
Stomach	Ren 12	Zhong Wan
Spleen	Liver 13	Zhang Men
Heart	Ren 14	Ju Que
Small Intestine	Ren 4	Guan Yuan
Bladder	Ren 3	Zhong Ji
Kidney	GB 25	Jing Men
Pericardium	Ren 17	Tan Zhong
San Jiao	Ren 5	Shi Men
Gallbladder	GB 24	Ri Yue
Liver	Liver 14	Qi Men

Classical acupuncture point function guidance is combined with needling techniques, which include the nine needles theory to determine how to treat the mu points, as well as all acupuncture points. The central guidance is a reinforcing or reducing technique that can be applied with a device to create the reinforcing or reducing influence (movement in the body/channels), which is the approach for all acupuncture points, including the mu points. The mu points are local points for treating the internal organs; they are also destination points. When treating an internal organ, the mu points can be treated.

---

6   Yang, C. (2004) *A Systematic Classic of Acupuncture and Moxibustion*. Boulder, CO: Blue Poppy Press.

The mu points are used as a diagnostic method to determine imbalances of the internal organs. Mu points are in close proximity to an organ and the condition of the organ can appear at the mu acupuncture points.

Transporting points

Wu Xing

The five transporting points are presented in the *Ling Shu*, Chapter 2, "The Roots of the Acupuncture Points," and their five aspects of physiology are presented in the *Ling Shu*, Chapter 44, "The Smooth Flowing Qi Divides One Day into Four Seasons," as well as in many chapters in the *Nei Jing*. We begin with the *Nei Jing* presentation of the five transporting points and then introduce *Nan Ching* theories.

> Huangdi asked: I have heard there are five different applications of the Five Shu points; could you tell me about them? Qibo answered: There are five organs in the human body. Each Zang organ relates to five aspects of physiology (which are seasons, days, colors, tones and tastes).[7]

Table 7.4 contains the five transporting acupuncture points. Notice there are no five phases. Table 7.5 contains the five aspects of physiology of the five transporting acupuncture points.

This is how to read Table 7.4:

- Well points treat any condition of the internal organs. Spring points treat changes in complexion. Stream points treat conditions that change from time to time. River points treat changes in the voice. Sea points treat diseases of the stomach from diet and local blood stagnation. The practitioner would identify the imbalanced channel/organ and

---

7   Wang, Z. & Wang, J. (2007) *Ling Shu Acupuncture*. Irvine, CA: Ling Shu Press.

CLINICAL POINT SELECTION

then treat the corresponding point that treats the conditions listed.

- Follow the same approach for the remaining correspondences/physiology: treat the well points on the Kidney channel for any condition in the winter, treat the stream point on the Heart channel for any condition during the summer, and so on.

Note there are no five-phases points (five-elements points) in the *Nei Jing*; these are introduced in the *Nan Ching*. There is also no zangfu pattern differential with the five transporting points in the *Nei Jing*.

A reinforcing or reducing technique is applied based on the diagnosis.

Table 7.4: Transporting acupuncture points

Yin channels	Jing Well	Ying Spring	Shu Stream	Jing River	He Sea
Lung	11	10	9	8	5
Spleen	1	2	3	5	9
Heart	9	8	7	4	3
Kidney	1	2	3	7	10
Pericardium	9	8	7	5	3
Liver	1	2	3	4	8

Yang channels	Jing Well	Ying Spring	Shu Stream	Jing River	He Sea
Large Intestine	1	2	3	5	11
Stomach	45	44	43	41	36
Small Intestine	1	2	3	5	8
Bladder	67	66	65	60	40
San Jiao	1	2	3	6	10
Gallbladder	44	43	41	38	34

ACUPUNCTURE POINT CATEGORIES IN THE HAN DYNASTY

Table 7.5: *Nei Jing* transporting points and five aspects of physiology

Nei Jing	Well	Spring	Stream	River	Sea
	Jing	Ying	Shu	Jing	He
	Treats zang diseases Treats all organ conditions	Changes in color (facial complexion)	Conditions that change from time to time	Changes in the voice	Stomach disease Diseases related to diet Blood stagnation in the superficial collaterals
Organ	Kidney	Liver	Heart	Spleen	Lung
Season	Winter	Spring	Summer	Long Summer	Fall
Days (Stems)	Ren Gui	Jia Yi	Bing Ding	Wu Ji	Geng Xin
Colors	Black	Green	Red	Yellow	White
Tastes	Salty	Sour	Bitter	Sweet	Pungent
Tone	Yu	Jiao	Zhen	Gong	Shang

The *Nan Ching* (*Classic of Difficulties*) and five-phases acupuncture points

The *Nan Ching* (*Classic of Difficulties*) presents the five-phases acupuncture points, overlaid on the *Nei Jing* five transporting points. For the first time, there are five-phases points located on the acupuncture channels.

Nan Ching, Chapter 68, presents the most common theory used in modern clinical practice:

> Difficulty Sixty-eight says: The five viscera and six bowels all have wells, brooks, streams, rivers, and uniting [points]. What [illnesses] do these places all govern?
>
> Answer: The Classic says the place of exiting makes for the

wells, the place of flowing makes for the brooks, the place of pouring makes for the streams, the place of movement makes for the rivers, and the place of entering makes for the uniting [points].

The well rules fullness below the heart. The brooks rule bodily heat. The streams rule bodily heaviness and joint pain. The rivers rule panting and coughing, cold and heat. And the uniting [points] rule counterflow qi and discharge [or diarrhea]. These are the five viscera and six bowels, wells, brooks, streams, river, and the uniting [points] places and the diseases they govern.[8]

Brooks are also called spring points.

Note that there is no acupuncture theory supporting those functions in the chapter. Table 7.7 is an attempt to provide a five phases logic to support the functions, it contains the element (phase), organ and channel relationship. Table 7.6 contains the five phases with the five transporting acupuncture points.

Table 7.6: Five transporting and five-phases acupuncture points

Yin Channels	Wood Jing Well	Fire Ying Spring	Earth Shu Stream	Metal Jing River	Water He Sea
Lung	11	10	9 T	8 H	5 S
Spleen	1	2 T	3 H	5 S	9
Heart	9 T	8 H	7 S	4	3
Kidney	1 S	2	3	7 T	10 H
Pericardium	9 T	8 H	7 S	5	3
Liver	1 H	2 S	3	4	8 T

---

8   Flaws, B. (2009) *The Classic of Difficulties: A Translation of the Nan Jing.* Boulder, CO: Blue Poppy Press

ACUPUNCTURE POINT CATEGORIES IN THE HAN DYNASTY

Yang Channels	Metal Jing Well	Water Ying Spring	Wood Shu Stream	Fire Jing River	Earth He Sea
Large Intestine	1 H	2 S	3	5	11 T
Stomach	45 S	44	43	41 T	36 H
Small Intestine	1	2	3 T	5 H	8 S
Bladder	67 T	66 H	65 S	60	40
San Jiao	1	2	3 T	6 H	10 S
Gallbladder	44	43 T	41 H	38 S	34

Code:

T = Tonification acupuncture point is the parent phase acupuncture point

S = Sedation acupuncture point is the child phase acupuncture point

H = Horary acupuncture point is the same phase as the channel phase

Nan Ching five-phases functions and explanation

Table 7.7 contains a five-phases logic that attempts to explain the *Nan Ching* functions of the five-phases acupuncture points.

This is how to read Table 7.7:

Example: Treating wood—Liver/Gallbladder

Metal controls wood, for example the Lung channel controls the Liver channel. The metal acupuncture point controls the wood channel/organ. The wood acupuncture point strongly influences a wood channel, which is its own five-phases channel—it is a horary acupuncture point. A horary acupuncture point is the acupuncture point which is the same phase as the channel element. Liver 1 is the wood acupuncture point on the Liver channel, and Gallbladder 41

79

CLINICAL POINT SELECTION

is the wood acupuncture point on the Gallbladder channel—they can strongly influence the channel. It is the *needling technique* that determines whether reinforcing or reducing occurs in the body, as well as the magnitude or strength of the influence. If metal is reinforced it controls the wood by containing it. If metal is reduced it reduces the normal force that is controlling wood; it is usually applied for a wood deficient condition to allow wood to grow. Wood channels are reduced when there is an excess and reinforced when there is a deficiency. The channel phase relationships and the reinforcing and reducing needling techniques would be combined in the future to become part of the four-needle acupuncture method.

The controller and horary point are reinforced or reduced to match the treatment plan, which shows that every acupuncture point can be reinforced or reduced. The needling technique determines what occurs in a treatment, not a five-phases relationship between an acupuncture point and a channel, nor a channel-to-channel five-phases relationship.

Yin channel well acupuncture points are wood, and Yang well acupuncture points are metal. Metal treats wood by the controlling relationship and wood treats (influences) wood by being a horary phase. In this example, the well acupuncture points on the Yin and Yang channel both treat the Liver-Gallbladder channel and the epigastrium. The needling technique of reinforcing or reducing is applied based on the treatment plan.

Yin channel spring acupuncture points are fire, and Yang channel spring acupuncture points are water; water controls fire and fire treats fire, both treat febrile (heat) conditions. The needling technique determines if a reinforcing or reducing action occurs. That five-phases logic is extended to all the transporting five-phases points.

The basic five-phases theory is a narrow acupuncture theory when it is applied to the five transporting points, as it identifies one point to treat specific symptoms. The five phases are used to identify one acupuncture point to treat for an elemental excess or deficiency.

Actually, it's a mixture of narrow and wide. It's narrow as one point is selected, the parent or child phase (element) point, but it treats any excess or deficiency, it is not pattern or pathogen limited, but treats any pattern and pathogen of an organ/element. It is a wide theory from that viewpoint. It is an example that acupuncture reduces the entire channel/organ, and reinforces the channel/organ.

The basic five-phases approach to acupuncture point selection implies that one acupuncture point reinforces or reduces the channel better than any other acupuncture point. *Nan Ching*'s five-phases theory has become the predominant theory for applying the transporting acupuncture points in clinical practice. A channel-based approach to creating acupuncture treatments includes the five-phases theory, as well as other theories that offer a variety of options for creating acupuncture treatments.

Table 7.7: Nan Ching five-phases functions and explanation

	Well	Spring	Stream	River	Sea
Yang channels	Metal	Water	Wood	Fire	Earth
Five-phases relationship	Controlling element	Controlling element	Controlling element	Controlling element	Controlling element
Organ	**Liver**	**Heart**	**Spleen**	**Lungs**	**Kidneys**
Condition	Fullness in the heart, (which includes the epigastrium)	Febrile Heat	Damp (heavy sensation, joint pain)	Panting, cough (considered asthma too)	Counter-flow qi, discharge, diarrhea Water
Yin channels	Wood	Fire	Earth	Metal	Water
Five-phases relationship	Horary phase	Horary phase	Horary phase	Horary phase	Horary phase

CHAPTER 8

Treating Organs

Shang Hang Lun (*SHL*) is a classic herbal book on Chinese herbal formulas. It is one of the oldest Chinese herbal traditions. *SHL* is interesting because it is a book of herbal formulas that was unlike the earliest Ben Cao tradition, which began as a pharmacopeia of individual herbs and only developed well-known and popular herbal formulas in later years. Herbal formulas are a group of individual herbs that combine to create a healing effect greater than individual herbs. Acupuncture can also work in that way. Treating acupuncture points (or areas) on a channel and treating supporting channels provides a synergistic effect that cannot be obtained with just a single acupuncture point. Where Chinese herbal medicine developed into a sophisticated herbal formula medicine, clinical point selection (acupuncture point combinations) didn't develop in a similar way. Transitioning from a point-driven approach to a channel/area-driven one is essential in understanding the synergy created in a channel-based approach to acupuncture.

Acupuncture point selection is commonly taught as a single-point method in Chinese medical schools: a list of conditions each point treats is presented to give the reader the idea that each point can actually treat all the conditions. This method of organizing acupuncture points disconnects any understanding of how treating points stimulates a channel and everything along the trajectory, which leads the student to believe the two are not one, preventing a synergy in creating acupuncture channel-point combinations.

The goal for treatment is to stimulate the body via channels to remove excesses or guide Qi to reinforce an organ and area. The amount of stimulation necessary to obtain the clinical goal varies based on the condition of the patient; in general, less is better. Developing a treatment plan with minimal areas of treatment is the starting point. Following guidance from the *Ling Shu*—checking the response of the patient—determines if additional treatment is necessary. For example, if the source point on a channel is treated to tonify the Spleen, checking the pulse after a few minutes will indicate whether the body is responding. If the pulse does not move toward becoming a normal pulse, it is advised to add other areas on the channel for treatment or add a supporting channel. With experience, the practitioner can effectively determine the severity of the condition, the health of the patient and the number of points and channels to treat.

Framework for treatment

The goal of treatment is to stimulate points and areas to achieve the therapeutic effect. The level of stimulation is the key to clinical effectiveness. Stimulation includes the number of points treated, their insertion sequence and the strength of the reinforcing or reducing technique. A beginning step in this treatment process is to think of treating one area or point; if that is not effective, then try two or more areas of stimulation. The following is a framework (the areas/points to be treated should be adjusted based on the unique condition of each patient) for this channel-based treatment approach:

1. Treat the stream point alone.
2. Treat the sea point alone.
3. Treat the stream and sea points together.
4. Treat the mu or shu point alone.

5. Treat the stream and mu or shu points.

6. Treat the sea and mu or shu points.

7. Treat the stream, sea and mu or shu points.

Treating the stream or sea point alone can always be performed first before using the two- or three-point combinations. Your experience will guide whether to begin with a one-, two- or three-point combination.

The foundation point combination to treat an organ is the stream and sea points on the imbalanced channel. That combination can be used for a low to moderate condition. For a more serious condition, treat the stream, sea and then the front mu or back shu point. Generally, the two or three acupuncture point combinations stimulate the channel more effectively than one point; the points in these combinations are some of the most common points used in clinical practice. This approach is flexible, so include other acupuncture points that fit the clinical condition. Try the suggested point and combinations presented to gain a base for its effectiveness. It is important to be guided by the reality that we treat the channel by way of points and areas along it.

Treatment sequence

One of the most important aspects of an acupuncture treatment is the sequence of the treatment; that is, the exact order in which the needles are inserted. The sequence of treatment is different for a reinforcing or reducing technique. The examples here show the sequences.

Reinforcing begins at the most distal area in the treatment and moves toward the destination—for example, Kidney 3 and then Bladder 23 to reinforce the Kidneys, or Spleen 6, Spleen 9 and then Liver 13 to reinforce the Spleen.

Reducing begins where the condition is located and moves

away from that area to distal areas—for example, Liver 14 and then Liver 2 to reduce the Liver, or Stomach 21 and then Stomach 44 to reduce the Stomach.

Destination

I created the name *destination point*™ to describe the location in which a reinforcing treatment is directed. For instance, if there is Spleen qi deficiency, the plan is to reinforce the Spleen, which means increasing the circulation of Qi into the Spleen. Liver 13 is the mu point of the Spleen, and needling that point at the end of the treatment directs the treatment (Qi) to the Spleen. Designing a treatment to end at the destination area is the most direct way to influence a targeted area. I often joke, "I am not in the hope business" in the sense that we have thousands of years of successfully treating conditions using acupuncture skill; we don't simply insert needles and hope there is clinical effectiveness. It requires a lot of hoping to think that needling Kidney 3 alone moves Qi to the Kidneys to tonify, energize and restore them. In my experience, treating Kidney 3, Kidney 10 and then Gallbladder 25 (front mu point of the Kidneys) is much more effective in influencing the Kidneys, and patients often feel the Qi flow (a sensation) through the pathway being treated to the organ. The feeling that the patient experiences is a significant signal to both the patient and practitioner—it confirms that the treatment is working as it is intended to.

The objective for creating acupuncture treatments is to stimulate the body by stimulating channels to achieve the therapeutic effect. Tables 8.1–8.7 list the foundation acupuncture point combinations to treat the internal organs. Every health condition can be categorized from moderate to severe. The practitioner's experience can determine the levels, using a scale of 1–10 as a guide (2–4 is mild to moderate, 5–7 is moderate to strong and 8–10 is strong to severe). For a mild condition, try one point or area of treatment, and add more if necessary.

Treating organs

Tables 8.1–8.7 contain a variety of acupuncture point combinations. The acupuncture point combinations range from mild to strong to severe deficient and excess conditions.

Reinforcing sequence for moderate to strong deficient conditions

Table 8.1 contains a reinforcing sequence for moderate to strong deficient conditions. The acupuncture point combinations include stream and sea acupuncture points. Select one or both of the points.

Table 8.1: Stream and sea acupuncture point combinations

Sequence	1	2
Channel/Organ	Stream	Sea
Lung	Lung 9	Lung 5
Large Intestine	Large Intestine 3	Large Intestine 11
Stomach	Stomach 43	Stomach 36
Spleen	Spleen 3	Spleen 9
Heart	Heart 7	Heart 3
Small Intestine	Small Intestine 3	Small Intestine 8
Bladder	Bladder 65	Bladder 40
Kidney	Kidney 3	Kidney 10
Pericardium	Pericardium 7	Pericardium 3
San Jiao	San Jiao 3	San Jiao 10
Gallbladder	Gallbladder 41	Gallbladder 34
Liver	Liver 3	Liver 8

Deficiency examples:

- Liver deficiency: treat Liver 3 and Liver 8 for any deficiency of the Liver.

CLINICAL POINT SELECTION

- Spleen deficiency: treat Spleen 3 and Spleen 9 for any deficiency of the Spleen.
- Kidney deficiency: treat Kidney 3 and Kidney 10 for any deficiency of the Kidneys.

Reinforcing sequence for treating intense (severe) deficient conditions

Table 8.2 contains a reinforcing sequence for treating intense (severe) deficient conditions. The acupuncture point combinations include stream, sea and the front mu *or* back shu acupuncture point combinations. Select two or more of the points.

Table 8.2: Stream, sea and mu/shu acupuncture point combinations

Sequence	1	2	3	3
Organ	Stream	Sea	Front mu	Back shu
Lung	Lung 9	Lung 5	Lung 1	Bladder 13
Large Intestine	Large Intestine 3	Large Intestine 11	Stomach 25	Bladder 25
Stomach	Stomach 43	Stomach 36	Ren 12	Bladder 21
Spleen	Spleen 3	Spleen 9	Liver 13	Bladder 20
Heart	Heart 7	Heart 3	Ren 14	Bladder 15
Small Intestine	Small Intestine 3	Small Intestine 8	Ren 4	Bladder 27
Bladder	Bladder 65	Bladder 40	Ren 3	Bladder 28
Kidney	Kidney 3	Kidney 10	Gallbladder 25	Bladder 23
Pericardium	Pericardium 7	Pericardium 3	Ren 17	Bladder 14
San Jiao	San Jiao 3	San Jiao 10	Ren 5	Bladder 22
Gallbladder	Gallbladder 41	Gallbladder 34	Gallbladder 24	Bladder 19
Liver	Liver 3	Liver 8	Liver 14	Bladder 18

Example: Treat Spleen 3, Spleen 9 and then Liver 13 for any deficiency of the Spleen.

Reducing sequence for moderate to strong excess conditions

Table 8.3 contains a reducing sequence for moderate to strong excess conditions. The acupuncture point combinations include sea and stream acupuncture points. Select one or both of the points.

Table 8.3: Stream and sea acupuncture point combinations

Sequence	1	2
Channel/Organ	Sea	Stream
Lung	Lung 5	Lung 9
Large Intestine	Large Intestine 11	Large Intestine 3
Stomach	Stomach 36	Stomach 43
Spleen	Spleen 9	Spleen 3
Heart	Heart 3	Heart 7
Small Intestine	Small Intestine 8	Small Intestine 3
Bladder	Bladder 40	Bladder 65
Kidney	Kidney 10	Kidney 3
Pericardium	Pericardium 3	Pericardium 7
San Jiao	San Jiao 10	San Jiao 3
Gallbladder	Gallbladder 34	Gallbladder 41
Liver	Liver 8	Liver 3

Example: Treat Gallbladder 34 and Gallbladder 41 for any excess in the Gallbladder.

Reducing sequence for strong and intense excess conditions

Table 8.4 contains a reducing sequence for strong and intense excess conditions. The acupuncture point combinations include mu or shu, sea and stream points. Select two or more of the points.

Table 8.4: Stream, sea, and mu or shu acupuncture point combinations

Sequence	1	1	2	3
Organ	Front mu	Back shu	Sea	Stream
Lung	Lung 1	Bladder 13	Lung 5	Lung 9
Large Intestine	Stomach 25	Bladder 25	Large Intestine 11	Large Intestine 3
Stomach	Ren 12	Bladder 21	Stomach 36	Stomach 43
Spleen	Liver 13	Bladder 20	Spleen 9	Spleen 3
Heart	Ren 14	Bladder 15	Heart 3	Heart 7
Small Intestine	Ren 4	Bladder 27	Small Intestine 8	Small Intestine 3
Bladder	Ren 3	Bladder 28	Bladder 40	Bladder 65
Kidney	Gallbladder 25	Bladder 23	Kidney 10	Kidney 3
Pericardium	Ren 17	Bladder 14	Pericardium 3	Pericardium 7
San Jiao	Ren 5	Bladder 22	San Jiao 10	San Jiao 3
Gallbladder	Gallbladder 24	Bladder 19	Gallbladder 34	Gallbladder 41
Liver	Liver 14	Bladder 18	Liver 8	Liver 3

Example: Treat Lung 1, Lung 5 and then Lung 9 for any excess of the Lung.

Acupuncture treatment strategy

Select channels first, then choose acupuncture points/areas for treatment. The areas can be acupuncture points, ashi areas or areas indicating pathology (e.g. areas with discoloration, swelling or sensitivity). The treatment areas should be reduced or reinforced. The following includes a variety of acupuncture point combination strategies:

1. Pick points from the same acupuncture point category or at the same anatomical level—for example, two stream points, two source points or two sea points. Stream and source points are near the ankle and the wrist, and sea points are near the knee and elbow.

2. The acupuncture needling sequence includes a few variations.

    - Needle points on the left side of the body and then needle points on the right side of the body. The practitioner decides whether to begin on the left or right side based on clinical experience. This is the recommended approach because it creates the strongest movement in a channel. Example: needle left Kidney 3 and then left Kidney 10, and then needle right Kidney 3 and then right Kidney 10.

    - Alternate left and right sides of the body point by point. Example: needle left Liver 3 and then right Liver 3, and then needle left Liver 8 and right Liver 8.

The variations of these treatments are listed in Tables 8.5 and 8.6. When there is a reinforcing method, apply the same principle for the reducing method sequence but reverse the order.

Ipsilateral sequence

The ipsilateral sequence is the preferred method for treating organs and channels. This approach generates the strongest circulation (movement) in a channel. Table 8.5 is a reinforcing sequence for the ipsilateral approach; treat one channel and then treat the paired channel.

CLINICAL POINT SELECTION

Table 8.5: Ipsilateral point combinations

Reinforcing sequence	1	2	1	2
	Left	Left	Right	Right
Channel/ Organ	Stream	Sea	Stream	Sea
Lung	Lung 9	Lung 5	Lung 9	Lung 5
Spleen	Spleen 3	Spleen 9	Spleen 3	Spleen 9
Heart	Heart 7	Heart 3	Heart 7	Heart 3
Kidney	Kidney 3	Kidney 10	Kidney 3	Kidney 10
Pericardium	Pericardium 7	Pericardium 3	Pericardium 7	Pericardium 3
Liver	Liver 3	Liver 8	Liver 3	Liver 8
Large Intestine	Large Intestine 3	Large Intestine 11	Large Intestine 3	Large Intestine 11
Stomach	Stomach 43	Stomach 36	Stomach 43	Stomach 36
Small Intestine	Small Intestine 3	Small Intestine 8	Small Intestine 3	Small Intestine 8
Bladder	Bladder 65	Bladder 40	Bladder 65	Bladder 40
San Jiao	San Jiao 3	San Jiao 10	San Jiao 3	San Jiao 10
Gallbladder	Gallbladder 41	Gallbladder 34	Gallbladder 41	Gallbladder 34

Alternating sequence

Table 8.6: Alternating point combinations

	1		2	
	Left	Right	Left	Right
Channel/ Organ	Stream	Stream	Stream	Stream
Lung-Large Intestine	Lung 9	Lung 9	Large Intestine 3	Large Intestine 3
Spleen-Stomach	Spleen 3	Spleen 3	Stomach 43	Stomach 43

Heart-Small Intestine	Heart 7	Heart 7	Small Intestine 3	Small Intestine 3
Kidney-Bladder	Kidney 3	Kidney 3	Bladder 65	Bladder 65
Pericardium-San Jiao	Pericardium 7	Pericardium 7	San Jiao 3	San Jiao 3
Liver-Gallbladder	Liver 3	Liver 3	Gallbladder 41	Gallbladder 41

Table 8.6: Alternating point combinations

	1	2	3	4
	Left	Right	Left	Right
Channel/Organ	Sea	Sea	Sea	Sea
Large Intestine-Lung	Large Intestine 11	Large Intestine 11	Lung 5	Lung 5
Stomach-Spleen	Stomach 36	Stomach 36	Spleen 9	Spleen 9
Small Intestine-Heart	Small Intestine 8	Small Intestine 8	Heart 3	Heart 3
Bladder-Kidney	Bladder 40	Bladder 40	Kidney 10	Kidney 10
San Jiao-Pericardium	San Jiao 10	San Jiao 10	Pericardium 3	Pericardium 3
Gallbladder-Liver	Gallbladder 34	Gallbladder 34	Liver 8	Liver 8

Table 8.6 contains the alternating reinforcing sequence method. This method is a common method applied in TCM. In this method, alternate treating stream points and then sea points on one side of the body and then the other side of the body. The reinforcing and reducing strategy guides the treatment sequence; for example, when reinforcing begin with stream points and then treat the sea points, and for a reducing strategy begin treating sea points and then treat the stream points.

Completion sequence

The completion method sequence is when the practitioner treats channels completely on one side of the body and then treats channels completely on the other side. Table 8.7 presents examples of the completion method. The examples treat the Yin-Yang paired channels on one side, and then the Yin-Yang paired channels on the other side.

Table 8.7: Completion point combinations

Sequence	1	2
	Left	Right
Channel	Stream, Sea	Stream, Sea
Lung	Lung 9, Lung 5, Large Intestine 3, Large Intestine 11	Lung 9, Lung 5, Large Intestine 3, Large Intestine 11
Spleen	Spleen 3, Spleen 9, Stomach 43, Stomach 36	Spleen 3, Spleen 9, Stomach 43, Stomach 36
Heart	Heart 7, Heart 3, Small Intestine 3, Small Intestine 8	Heart 7, Heart 3, Small Intestine 3, Small Intestine 8
Kidney	Kidney 3, Kidney 10, Bladder 65, Bladder 40	Kidney 3, Kidney 10, Bladder 65, Bladder 40
Pericardium	Pericardium 7, Pericardium 3, San Jiao 3, San Jiao 10	Pericardium 7, Pericardium 3, San Jiao 3, San Jiao 10
Liver	Liver 3, Liver 8, Gallbladder 41, Gallbladder 34	Liver 3, Liver 8, Gallbladder 41, Gallbladder 34

In addition to the acupuncture point combinations presented, the *Ling Shu* offers a two-point treatment that is very effective.

Ling Shu spring-stream points treatment

A two-point treatment is presented in Chapter 7 of the *Ling Shu*, "The Official Needles" and Chapter 24 of the *Ling Shu*, "The Receding [Qi] Diseases." The points are the spring and stream points. Treating two points in close proximity on the same channel can create a stronger influence than one point. If the condition is strong or stubborn in that the patient is not responding to treatments, consider a spring and stream point treatment.

In my experience, this approach can be applied to other areas of the body. For example, if there is a severely constrained Liver, treating both Liver 14 and Gallbladder 24—the mu points of the Liver and the Gallbladder—is very effective in releasing the condition.

Guidance

The treatment approaches presented in this chapter are a framework for treating organs and channels; this framework stimulates the channels and the body by treating common points used throughout the history of acupuncture. Including the correct needling sequence and the destination area adds a direct and powerful way to enhance the treatment by clearly directing the treatment to an area or by directly clearing away excesses. It is for the practitioner to determine if one, two, three or more points/areas require treatment.

A framework is a starting point for treatment. That starting point should change depending on the patient and their unique condition. The key is to maintain the principle: *treat the imbalanced channel directly with acupuncture points and areas*. The practitioner can add any of the acupuncture point categories—for instance, source, five transporting, mu, shu, lower he sea, luo, ashi—that fit the treatment plan. The goal is to learn how to most effectively influence the body to obtain the therapeutic effect. Measuring the effects of the acupuncture treatments while performing them and making adjustments during treatment involve clinically applying the insight of the ancient founders of acupuncture and will lead to increased clinical efficacy.

CHAPTER 9

Treating Emotions

Nei Jing marks a major shift in the practice of Chinese medicine. The shift is the movement away from theurgic medicine—the belief in supernatural intervention as a cause of illness. Early Chinese healing included the belief in ancestral medicine (curses of the ancestors) and later ghosts and demons as a cause of illness. *Nei Jing* includes a deep understanding of exogenous and endogenous pathogenic factors, lifestyle and the functioning of the human body. The compilers of *Nei Jing* began explaining a profound understanding of how those factors and activities influence health.

The *Su Wen* and *Ling Shu* medical texts present one of the first models for understanding the relationship between emotions and the human body—the body-mind relationship. Each text offers acupuncture theories to treat emotional disturbance, although it is more accurate to say that acupuncture can help release the intensity of charged emotional energy. Acupuncturists can potentially reduce or release the charged nature of emotions.

There are two main approaches for the diagnosis and treatment of emotional imbalance. The first is to identify and treat pathogens that may be involved in causing the imbalance, for example heat in the Heart can cause a Heart Shen disturbance, or Liver fire can disturb the Liver hun and activate anger and irritability. The second treatment approach is based on life dynamics that influence the psychological and emotional state of a person; that influence most often originates within family dynamics and required societal interaction (conditioning). Conditioning results from being continually exposed to unfavorable emotional influences, for instance dysfunctional parents or unfavorable school environments that have potent effects on a child's emotional and psychological well-being. Leaving unfavorable environments and receiving professional assistance from a mental health professional is often crucial. A skilled acupuncturist can have a powerful effect in releasing emotional imbalances and charged emotional energy. The image of puncturing a balloon to release air is similar to releasing charged emotional energy. For the acupuncturist, strategically treating channels and points can bring powerful emotional relief to a person.

Chinese medicine includes the five-Shen model for understanding emotional imbalances. That model is one of the earliest medical insights about the mind-body relationship; it is based on the inseparable nature of the internal organs and their related psycho-emotional qualities. The five-Shen model is not described completely in any one chapter in the *Su Wen* or *Ling Shu*. Instead, a comprehensive understanding needs to be pieced together from Chinese medical classics, Chinese philosophy and Daoist teachings. This chapter contains essential information about the five Shen that provides the basis to make a five-Shen diagnosis and treat accordingly.

A diamond in the rough

A diamond in the rough is an image I use that illustrates how life's stressors influence a person. Each person has a diamond, which is his or her Shen (i.e. spirit or true nature). The rough includes the stressors, conditioning, imprints, patterns, emotions and unfavorable influences that exist in life. The rough parts of life can cause emotional disturbance with varying degrees of intensity. During times of emotional imbalance, our attention is on the rough and away from our spirit, causing expression of the rough in our life;

roughness includes emotional turmoil. Because roughness is not our true nature, we can let it go, but letting go seems to be very challenging for some people. Acupuncture can assist in helping a person let go of what they do not need, and when a person lets go of what they do not need they often become aware of their spirit. That awareness can be a life-changing experience in the sense that a person becomes conscious of an aspect of themselves that is not their common state of consciousness. When we are conscious of our true nature it can inspire living a life that allows that consciousness to be our natural, normal way of living.

The five Shen

The *Su Wen* and *Ling Shu* present the qualities of each of the five Shen, which provide the basis for a five-Shen diagnosis. The main qualities or resonances are from Chapter 8 in the *Ling Shu*, "Roots and Spirit," and Chapter 5 in the *Su Wen*, "The Manifestation of Yin and Yang from the Macrocosm to the Microcosm." I have summarized the information in the following tables. Instead of identifying the imbalanced channel(s), the imbalanced Shens are identified. The information about the five Shen listed below comprises a diagnostic model that is used to identify the imbalanced Shen(s).

Table 9.1: Five-Shen resonances

Organ	The five Shen and their inherent qualities
Heart	The Heart is the sovereign of all organs and represents the consciousness of one's spirit. It is responsible for intelligence, wisdom and spiritual transformation.
Liver	The Liver is like the general; it is intelligent and courageous.
Lung	The Lung is the advisor; it helps the heart in regulating the Qi.
Kidneys	The Kidneys store vitality, which mobilizes the four extremities. The Kidneys also benefit the memory and willpower.
Spleen	The Stomach and Spleen are like warehouses; they store food and essences. They digest, transform and transport food and nutrients.

Table 9.2: The five storehouses

Organ	The five storehouses
Heart	The Heart is the storehouse for the channels; it is the shelter of the spirit (Shen spirit).
Liver	The Liver is the storehouse of blood; it is the shelter of the human soul (hun spirit).
Lung	The Lung is the storehouse of Qi; it is the shelter of the animal spirit (po spirit).
Kidneys	The Kidneys are the storehouse of the seminal essence; they are the shelter of the will (zhi spirit).
Spleen	The Spleen is the storehouse of nourishment; it is the shelter of thought (yi spirit).

Table 9.3: The five Yin organs

Organ	The five Yin organs
Heart	The spirit of the Heart is called the Shen; it rules mental and creative functions.
Liver	The spirit of the Liver is called the hun; it rules the nervous system and gives rise to extra-sensory awareness.
Lung	The spirit of the Lung is called the po; it rules the animalistic instincts and physical strength and endurance.
Kidneys	The spirit of the Kidneys is called the zhi; it rules the will, drive, ambition and survival instinct.
Spleen	The spirit of the Spleen is known as the yi; it rules logic and rational thought.

Table 9.4: The five Shen and emotions

Organ	The five Shen and emotions
Heart	Heart and Small Intestine Too much joy can cause a depletion of the Heart qi. A Heart Shen imbalance can cause a loss of identity and a loss of purpose in life. Trauma can cause a Shen disturbance and a Shen imbalance. Emotional imbalance of any of the five Shen can also influence the Heart Shen. Imbalances of the Heart Shen can manifest as hastiness, impatience, arrogance, cruelty and hatred.

Liver	Liver and gallbladder Anger can injure the liver. Imbalances of the Liver and the hun can manifest as anger, irritability, frustration and repression.
Lung	Lung and Large Intestine Extreme grief can injure the Lung. Imbalances of the Lungs and the po can manifest as grief, sadness, sorrow, isolation, loneliness and inability to forgive.
Kidneys	Kidneys and Bladder Fear and fright will damage the Kidneys. Imbalances of the Kidneys and the zhi can manifest as fear, fright, paranoia and lack of willpower.
Spleen	Spleen and Stomach Excessive worry will deplete Spleen qi. Imbalances of the Spleen and the yi can manifest as pensiveness, worry, and obsessive and repetitive thinking.

Table 9.5: The five Shen, emotions and five-phase interactions

Organ	The five Shen, emotions and five-phase interactions
Heart	Too much joy can cause a depletion of the Heart qi. This can be counterbalanced by fear. Water controls fire. The zhi controls the Shen.
Liver	Anger can injure the Liver, but sadness can relieve anger. Metal controls wood. The po controls the hun.
Lung	Extreme grief can injure the Lung, but it may be countered by the emotion of happiness. Fire controls metal. The Shen controls the po.
Kidneys	Fear and fright will damage the Kidneys. They can be defeated with understanding, logic and rational thinking. Earth controls water. The yi controls the zhi.
Spleen	Excessive worry will deplete Spleen qi, but anger can restrain this worry. Wood controls earth. The hun controls the yi.

The five phases controlling relationships listed in Table 9.5 may be a source for the use of the controlling cycle in the four-needle five-element acupuncture method.

The following quote from Chapter 8 of the *Ling Shu*, "Roots and Spirit," provides insight into how to evaluate the impact of fright, stress and anxiety: "When the heart and mind is frightened and full of distressed thoughts and anxiety, it can result in injury to the spirit. This can result in fear and loss of self."[1]

This quote can be interpreted in the following way: with stress and emotional turmoil, we can lose awareness and connection to self (i.e. spirit). Acupuncture can assist in clearing or releasing the emotionally charged energy that is unfavorably influencing a person. Acupuncture can also assist in creating the opportunity for awareness of self and Shen.

Treatment strategy

There are a few approaches for treating emotions and Shen imbalances:

- Reduce the excess and excessiveness in the channel/organ and five Shen.
- Reinforce an organ/Shen to allow the natural quality within that five Shen to be expressed. When an organ is deficient, a person can express the unfavorable emotions.
- Attune or align to Shen. Treating channels and points that relate to shen can guide a person's focus, attention and awareness to the Shen.

Any variation and combination of the three approaches can be applied in a treatment or series of treatments.

A diagnosis and treatment plan should include the following:

- Identify the emotions the patient is experiencing.
- Identify the Shen and organ related to the emotions.
- Directly treat the organs/channels/Shen that are imbalanced.

---

[1] Wu, J. (2002) *Ling Shu or The Spiritual Pivot*. Hawaii: University of Hawaii Press.

With many people, emotional imbalances occur due to excess, which requires a reducing treatment approach. A strategy for treatment begins with matching emotions to their corresponding Shen and organ. In the metaphor of the diamond in the rough, imbalances of these emotions are the rough, and acupuncture (and pricking to bleed) can assist in clearing the roughness, revealing the shining light of the diamond (i.e. the Shen). Awareness of your Shen can inspire, motivate and provide the incentive for change and transformation.

Treating emotional imbalances and the five Shen

There are a few approaches to treat emotional imbalances. One way to differentiate treatment is by the severity of the emotions—how intense they are. Measuring the severity can be done on a scale of 1–10. Experience will guide the practitioner in determining the levels.

The sequence of needle insertion is very important in treatment. Tables 9.6–9.10 present my recommended acupuncture points and treatment sequences; they can be used as presented or as the basis for treatments developed to treat the unique condition of each patient.

The following are basic calm-the-Shen treatments.

Option 1

1. Du 24
2. Yintang
3. Pericardium 6, Liver 3

Table 9.6. contains four acupuncture points that comprise a basic calm-the-Shen-treatment. That treatment can be applied in most treatments.

CLINICAL POINT SELECTION

Table 9.6: Du 24, Yintang, Pericardium 6, and Liver 3 point combination

	1	2	
1	Du 24	Yintang	Treat Du 24 first and then Yintang. Du 24 is needled transverse backward. Use ½ cun needle on both points.
2	PC 6	Liver 3	Treat Pericardium 6 first then Liver 3. There are two main sequence options that can be applied: the first is same sided and the second is diagonal. The same-sided treatment is Pericardium 6 then Liver 3 on the right or left side, then repeat on the opposite side. Diagonal needling is treating left Pericardium 6, right Liver 3, right Pericardium 6, and then left Liver 3. Use your experience to determine on which side to begin the treatment. My preference is to needle Pericardium 6 transverse toward the fingers and needle Liver 3 oblique toward the toes in both sequences.

The first part of this treatment is Du 24 and Yintang, and they should be needled in that order. That acupuncture point combination is a local treatment to calm the mind. The second part of the treatment is Pericardium 6 and Liver 3. This treatment should follow that sequence. That acupuncture point combination reduces the Liver (Liver qi stagnation) and calms the Shen by reducing the Pericardium, which reduces excess in the Heart Shen.

Option 2

When a stronger calm-the-Shen treatment is needed, add Gallbladder 13 to Du 24, Yintang, Pericardium 6 and Liver 3.

Table 9.7: Du 24, Gallbladder 13 and Yintang point combination

Shen	Influences all Shen	Influences all Shen	Influences all Shen
	1	2	3
Po	Du 24	Gallbladder 13	Yintang
Po	Du 24	Gallbladder 13	Yintang
Yi	Du 24	Gallbladder 13	Yintang

Yi	Du 24	Gallbladder 13	Yintang
Shen	Du 24	Gallbladder 13	Yintang
Shen	Du 24	Gallbladder 13	Yintang
Zhi	Du 24	Gallbladder 13	Yintang
Zhi	Du 24	Gallbladder 13	Yintang
Hun	Du 24	Gallbladder 13	Yintang
Hun	Du 24	Gallbladder 13	Yintang

Gallbladder 13 can be specific to the Liver and Gallbladder and the hun, as well as being a systemic calm-the-Shen influence as a local treatment, meaning it is not limited to a pattern. The name of Gallbladder 13 is *Ben Shen* ("mind root") and it has a strong calming effect, regardless of the cause of the distress.

Example:

1. Du 24

2. Gallbladder 13

3. Yintang

4. Pericardium 6, Liver 3

The acupuncture points should be treated in the exact order listed above. It is a two-part treatment: part one treats Du 24, then Gallbladder 13 on each side and then Yintang; part two treats Pericardium 6 and then Liver 3.

Option 3

Below are calm-the-Shen treatments that you can use when organs (Shen) are involved or the condition is chronic or acute. This approach targets specific channels/organs based on the imbalanced emotions and their relationship to the five Shen.

This treatment is Du 24, Gallbladder 13 and Yintang, plus a mu *or* shu acupoint and a luo point. *Nei Jing* states that the five Shen are stored in the yin organs; when a mu and shu point is reduced it clears excesses in the organ that contribute to emotional imbalances. Luo points and luo collaterals are buffers that hold pathogens, including emotionally charged energy. Treating the luo points and collaterals releases the emotionally charged energy. Table 9.8 contains the mu, shu and luo points combinations. Select a mu *or* shu point.

Table 9.8: Mu/shu and luo point combination

Shen	Organ	Front mu	Back shu	Luo point
		1	1	2
Po	Lung	Lung 1	Bladder 13	Lung 7
Po	Large Intestine	Stomach 25	Bladder 25	Large Intestine 6
Yi	Stomach	Ren 12	Bladder 21	Stomach 40
Yi	Spleen	Liver 13	Bladder 20	Spleen 4
Shen	Heart	Ren 14	Bladder 15	Heart 5
Shen	Small Intestine	Ren 4	Bladder 27	Small Intestine 7
Zhi	Bladder	Ren 3	Bladder 28	Bladder 58
Zhi	Kidney	Gallbladder 25	Bladder 23	Kidney 4
Hun	Gallbladder	Gallbladder 24	Bladder 19	Gallbladder 37
Hun	Liver	Liver 14	Bladder 18	Liver 5

Example:

1. Du 24, Gallbladder 13, Yintang
2. Right Liver 14 and then right Liver 5
3. Left Liver 14 and then left Liver 5

Option 4

The mu or shu and luo points combination can be effective, and sometimes a stronger treatment is necessary for very strong and intense emotional conditions. In that case, it is very effective to add points on the head and leg (which is metaphorically called treating heaven and earth: heaven is the head and earth is the leg). Table 9.9 adds two sets of points on the head and leg: Stomach 8 and Stomach 40, and Gallbladder 13 and Gallbladder 37. This treatment adds a head and luo point to option 3 when the hun (Liver-Gallbladder) and the yi (Spleen-Stomach) are involved in the condition. A hun and yi imbalance is stress influencing digestion, anger stimulating worry, and wood overacting on earth; it is one of the most common emotional imbalanced patterns.

Table 9.9: Stomach 8-Stomach 40 and then Gallbladder 13-Gallbladder 37 point combination

Shen	Organ	Head point heaven	Luo point leg
		1	2
Yi	Stomach	Stomach 8	Stomach 40
Yi	Spleen	Stomach 8	Stomach 40
Hun	Gallbladder	Gallbladder 13	Gallbladder 37
Hun	Liver	Gallbladder 13	Gallbladder 37

Example 1: Treating the Liver hun:

1. Du 24, Yintang
2. Right Gallbladder 13 and Gallbladder 37
3. Left Gallbladder 13 and Gallbladder 37

Example 2: Treating the Spleen yi:

1. Du 24, Yintang
2. Right Stomach 8 and then right Stomach 40
3. Left Stomach 8 and then left Stomach 40

Option 5

A way to treat any of the five Shen is to start with a basic calm-the-Shen treatment: Du 24 and Gallbladder 13, and then treat the luo

CLINICAL POINT SELECTION

point on the channel that is imbalanced. If the condition is strong and intense, add the luo points of the Yin-Yang channels being targeted. For example, use Liver 5 and Gallbladder 37 for treating emotional conditions related to the Liver hun.

Yintang can be added to any of the point combinations; it's a local calm-the-mind treatment that is not locked to a pattern. Imagine it is like puncturing a balloon to release the air. In this case, it's releasing emotionally charged energy.

Table 9.10: Du 24, Gallbladder 13 and luo points

Shen	Organ	Influences all Shen	Influences specific five Shen
		1	2
Po	Lung	Du 24, Gallbladder 13	Lung 7
Po	Large Intestine	Du 24, Gallbladder 13	Large Intestine 6
Yi	Stomach	Du 24, Gallbladder 13	Stomach 40
Yi	Spleen	Du 24, Gallbladder 13	Spleen 4
Shen	Heart	Du 24, Gallbladder 13	Heart 5
Shen	Small Intestine	Du 24, Gallbladder 13	Small Intestine 7
Zhi	Bladder	Du 24, Gallbladder 13	Bladder 58
Zhi	Kidney	Du 24, Gallbladder 13	Kidney 4
Hun	Gallbladder	Du 24, Gallbladder 13	Gallbladder 37
Hun	Liver	Du 24, Gallbladder 13	Liver 5

Example 1: Treating the Lung po:

1. Du 24
2. Gallbladder 13
3. Lung 7

Example 2: Treating the Heart Shen:

1. Du 24
2. Gallbladder 13
3. Small Intestine 7

Example 2 can be expanded. Consider Ren 17 and then Small Intestine 7, and if necessary add Small Intestine 4. A Yang channel's source point can strongly reduce a channel. A key function of Yang channels/organs is to empty; in this example, Small Intestine 4 is reduced to assist the luo point in clearing and emptying the excess emotionally charged energy; the reducing needling technique must be applied. Yang channel luo points can be added to a treatment to reduce a channel; they can be used alone or combined with other points.

Example 3: Alternative Heart Shen treatment:

1. Du 24
2. Gallbladder 13
3. Ren 17
4. Small Intestine 7
5. Small Intestine 4

The treatment is ipsilateral: right Small Intestine 7 and then right Small Intestine 4 and then the same two points on the left side. Your experience guides whether to begin on the right or left side.

For Spleen-Stomach-yi imbalances Stomach 8 can be added to the treatment.

From a Chinese medical viewpoint, treating emotions is treating the body-mind relationship. Releasing charged emotional energy (Qi) calms the body, mind and Shen. It must be stressed that the treatment approach and specific treatments presented do not change why a person suffers from emotional imbalances.

Professional mental health guidance should be considered when necessary; acupuncture is not a replacement for professional mental health care. Acupuncture can, however, reduce the influence, allowing the person to look at themselves and others in a different way, which can change the unfavorable influence and their well-being.

Chinese medicine contains theories and principles that guide the practitioner to *customize* treatments for each patient. The treatment approaches in this chapter are a framework which can be applied alone or as a base for creating treatments that best treat each patient. This framework is part of the Five-Shen model; practice working with the parts of the system to create the most effective treatments. Knowledge of the acupuncture channel system and the influences on the psychological condition of a person provides the basis for creating customized acupuncture treatments beyond the framework presented.

CHAPTER 10

Treating Pain

Pain is the most common condition treated with acupuncture. Chinese medicine offers a comprehensive understanding of pain and has multiple healing modalities for treatment. Applying an effective combination of modalities in treatment is key to obtaining the best clinical results possible.

Common causes of pain are repetitive movement, trauma and bi syndrome. Bi syndrome includes a variety of patterns that involve pathogens combined with damp: damp-wind, damp-cold, damp-heat and bone bi are common types. Bi syndrome also includes different types of arthritis. Treatment varies based on the specific nature of the pain condition reflected in a differential diagnosis. A common way to explain the treatment plan for pain is moving Qi and blood. *In reality, it is a sinew channel treatment which works on the musculoskeletal system.* Traditional sinew treatments include tuina (bodywork), acupuncture, moxibustion, cupping and topical liniments. Bodywork is a key to lasting effectiveness as it focuses on the origin of the condition; it should be performed before acupuncture to allow the treatment to work most effectively. Professional-level tuina includes orthopedic and physical therapy diagnosis and treatment methods.

The following eight Chinese medical modalities are effective for treating pain. Including two or more of these treatment methods can dramatically increase clinical effectiveness.

CLINICAL POINT SELECTION

1. Bodywork
2. Acupuncture
3. Moxa
4. Cupping
5. Liniments
6. Herbs
7. Exercise, medical qi gong, medical stretching/yoga
8. Electroacupuncture.

Pain treatment plan outline

1. Identify the problem area and channel; for pain it is usually the sinew channels, which includes the musculoskeletal system.
2. Determine the points and *areas* to treat; this includes a distal and local treatment plan. Use the most appropriate treatment variation: local, distal or distal and local combined.
3. Perform bodywork first.
4. Apply acupuncture.
5. Perform moxa while the needles are retained or after they are removed.
6. Apply cupping after needles are removed.
7. Apply liniments after the treatment and while at home.

Treatment principles

This section includes three main approaches for treating pain based on classical and traditional Chinese medicine. Each treatment should include one or more of the three approaches below.

1. The first approach is based on Chapter 13 of the *Ling Shu*, "The Conduits and their Sinews." This chapter presents treating the sinew channels, which contain the musculature system, by treating the painful points (ashi points); this is a local treatment.

2. The second approach includes a series of points that treat pain or bi syndrome. The points in this approach are stream and cleft points; one or both of the points can be included in the treatment. This is a distal treatment unless the condition is at the locations of those points.

3. The third approach is based on Chapter 25 of the *Su Wen*, "Following the Principle of Nature in Treating," and Chapter 7 of the *Ling Shu*, "Governing the Needles."

Chapter 25 of *Su Wen* presents what I call the *twelve-joint theory*, the basis for treating corresponding areas of the body based on joints and channels. "Man corresponds with nature; in heaven, there are Yin and Yang, in man there are the twelve large joints." "When one understands the principles of the twelve joints, even a sage will not surpass him."[1]

Chapter 7 of the *Ling Shu*, "Governing the Needles," is the basis for contralateral needling, specifically, the eighth needle: "The eight is called opposite needling. For this, one treats the right side when disease is on the left, and treats the left when disease in on the right."[2]

---

[1] Wu, N. & Wu, A. (2002) *Yellow Emperor's Canon of Internal Medicine*. Beijing: China Science Technology Press.
[2] Wu, J. (2002) *Ling Shu or The Spiritual Pivot*. Hawaii: University of Hawaii Press.

Those two chapters provide the foundation for contralateral acupuncture treatments. For a comprehensive understanding of this method of treatment, see my book *I Ching Acupuncture—The Balance Method*.

Treating the musculoskeletal system

Nei Jing presents five main channel systems of acupuncture. The practitioner should make a channel system diagnosis first—for example, the sinew channels or the main channels. Then the practitioner should identify the specific channels in that system—for instance, the foot Shaoyang sinew channel or the liver primary channel. Designating the channel system guides the treatment modalities to be applied in treatment; it also provides clarity for any other practitioners who may review patient records.

A sinew channel diagnosis and treatment should include a description similar to the following: stagnation in the foot Jueyin sinew channel; the diagnosis should not be Qi and blood stagnation in the Liver channel. The treatment plan can be to release stagnation in the foot Jueyin sinew channel (Liver). The action is to treat the sinew/muscle channels, not the primary channels. Treatment modalities correspond to the sinew channels, for example bodywork, moxa, cupping and liniments; the needling method is to needle into the muscles.

System 1

Treating musculoskeletal conditions

Local and distal treatments are the two main approaches for treating musculoskeletal conditions. An aspect of a distal treatment is evaluating the entire area of a channel to identify stagnations, blockages and imbalances that may exist between the local painful area and the most distal areas on the channel (that commonly is the well point); *often treating the in-between areas is essential for an effective treatment.*

1. Begin treatment with some form of bodywork to loosen muscles and release the locations of stagnation/blockage. Evaluate the entire sinew channel from beginning to end, and be sure to include the anatomical structures that influence the channel. For example, if there is pain on the foot Shaoyang sinew channel at Gallbladder 21 in the trapezius muscle, palpate at the neck at Gallbladder 20 and down the entire trapezius, rhomboids and para-spinal muscles on the back and then down the leg to the toes, following the foot Shaoyang sinew channel. The goal is to identify any blockages or imbalances on the channel and anatomical structures that contribute to the condition; the stagnated areas may be distal in the painful and stagnated areas.

    The *Ling Shu* provides guidance on how to identify areas to treat. Chapter 64 of the *Ling Shu*, "The Yin and Yang and the 25 Human Types," states the following:

    > One presses the fingers along the conduits and network [vessels] until they have reached a section that is rough with lumps. When there are knots blocking the passage, this will result in pain and blockage-illness all over the body. In serious cases, the movement is stopped, and this results in [sections that are] rough with lumps."[3]

    Another translation of this is as follows:

    > Closely follow the major channels of the body to see if they are congealed and rough, or tied up and obstructed. With all these, the body is painful with rheumatism.[4]

---

[3] Unschuld, P. (2016) *Huang Di Nei Jing Ling Shu: The Ancient Classic on Needle Therapy.* University of California Press.

[4] Wu, J. (2002) *Ling Shu or The Spiritual Pivot.* Hawaii: University of Hawaii Press.

The quotes above guide the practitioner to palpate the entire channel to identify obstructions, blockages, stagnations and knotted areas and to treat them directly. The practitioner should apply this approach when treating any type of pain.

2. The sinew channels are presented in every professional acupuncture text. Review them to view the exact areas the sinew/muscles flow. If you do not know their distribution, it may surprise you; for instance, the foot Yangming sinew channel (Stomach channel) flows to the spine—it can influence the spine, and those Stomach sinew channel areas on the spine can influence the areas of its distribution on the anterior of the body.

In general, if a muscle is involved in the condition, then needle into the muscle. It can be a transverse or oblique angle into the muscle. The goal is to release the muscle contraction, spasm or stagnation. A series of needles inserted at an oblique or transverse angle locally and in surrounding regions of the problem area is very effective in releasing muscles.

3. The treatment guidance above is a local treatment at the area of pain or imbalance. When areas of stagnation are identified and treated along the sinew channel a sinew channel can range from the foot to the neck, if the main pain is at the neck and there are also areas at the foot that are sore we can treat the areas at the foot too. We can treat two areas: the main pain at the neck and the soreness at the foot, treating the location of the foot is local to the foot.

4. Consider applying moxibustion during or after the acupuncture treatment.

5. Consider cupping after the needles are removed.

6. Consider using liniments and prescribing them for home use.

7. Consider herbs as part of the treatment.

System 2

Treating musculoskeletal conditions with stream and cleft points

In TCM, stream and cleft points are commonly treated for pain. System 2 can be used in conjunction with system 1 or used as a stand-alone treatment. Treat the stream or cleft point on the imbalanced channel. Stream and cleft points have traditionally been used for treating pain; one or both points can be treated. A rigid view can be that stream points treat a heavy sensation with pain—that is, damp and bi syndrome. Cleft points are presented as treating blood stagnation causing pain. In my experience, both points can treat pain of any etiology because they move the channel (Qi and blood); generally, my preference is to treat stream points.

Effectiveness test

A significant method for selecting effective distal points/areas is performing the "effectiveness test"™. I have developed this method to obtain immediate feedback as to whether a point or area will elicit pain relief. This test allows the practitioner to immediately know if a distal point is effective; therefore, it is not necessary to wait until the treatment is completed to obtain feedback.

The effectiveness test begins with identifying a distal point to treat pain. The method to make that selection can be one of the methods presented in this chapter or another method a practitioner includes in their practice. Press on the point or area. Do not just feel or gently touch the area, and do not palpate to identify a sensitive area, as this method does not use that approach. Press relatively strongly. The patient should feel the pressure; it does not have to be painful, but it must be more than a gentle touch. On a sensitivity scale of 1-10, around 2-3 would most likely be effective.

Practice and experience will guide the amount of pressure to exert. After a second or two, ask the patient if the pain is reduced. It is almost an immediate response; if it is, then needle it. If the pain is not reduced, try a different point (area) based on the methods in this book. If the points or areas on one side of the body are not effective, then apply the effectiveness test on the opposite side to which the test was applied.

Contralateral treatment is presented in *Ling Shu*, Chapter 7, "On Governing the Needles" and *Su Wen*, Chapter 5, "The Manifestation of Yin and Yang from the Macrocosm to the Microcosm." Some practitioners apply contralateral treatments in a narrow way, for example for treating luo collaterals pathology presented in *Su Wen*, Chapter 63, "Acupuncturing the Superficial Luo." *Ling Shu*, Chapter 7 and *Su Wen*, Chapter 5 do not present contralateral treatments connected to any pathology, pattern differential or specific condition; they are relationship based, both channel and anatomical imaging. Many practitioners have successfully treated patients with contralateral treatments based on anatomical (channel) relationships, for example the twelve joints. It is highly suggested you try it, and include the effectiveness test. Contralateral treatments can be applied alone or with same-sided treatments. Combining two or more approaches is part of the dosage of a treatment.

System 3: Twelve-joint theory

Method 1: Six-channel twelve-joint theory
Application 1
The twelve-joint theory is the source for a point-selection method for treating pain. This method involves anatomical and channel imaging, which includes the imaging of the six channels and the twelve joints. The six-channel anatomical relationships are the hand and foot, elbow and knee and the shoulder and hip. The twelve-joint theory includes the twelve main joints/anatomical

structures of the body and their relationship with each other. The twelve-joint theory relationships are as follows:

- Ankle and wrist
- Elbow and knee
- Should and hip.

The imaged paired channels treat each other—for instance, the ankle and wrist treat each other, meaning that pain at Gallbladder 40 can be treated at San Jiao 4, and Bladder 40 can treat pain at Small Intestine 8. This method combines the six-channel pairings at the twelve joints—foot and hand Shaoyang, and hand and foot Taiyang. Apply the effectiveness test on the six channels and the twelve joint locations first. Then, if necessary, apply the test around the corresponding area when the precise twelve-joint area does not reduce the pain level when applying the effectiveness test. Table 10.1 presents pairings and point combinations for this method.

Table 10.1: The twelve-joint theory

Six-channel pairs	Ankle and wrist	Knee and elbow	Hip and shoulder
Taiyang	Bladder 60 Small Intestine 4/5	Bladder 40 Small Intestine 8	Bladder 54 Small Intestine 10
Shaoyang	Gallbladder 40 San Jiao 4	Gallbladder 34 San Jiao 10	Gallbladder 29 San Jiao 14
Yangming	Stomach 41 Large Intestine 5	Stomach 35/36 Large Intestine 11	Stomach 30 Large Intestine 15
Taiyin	Spleen 5 Lung 9	Spleen 9 Lung 5	Spleen 12/13 Lung 2
Shaoyin	Kidney 3 Heart 7	Kidney 10 Heart 3	Kidney 11 Heart 1/Ashi
Jueyin	Liver 3 Pericardium 7	Liver 8 Pericardium 3	Liver 12 Pericardium 2

CLINICAL POINT SELECTION

Distal needling is the basis for this pain treatment. *My preference is to begin treatment on the contralateral side from the painful area.* The six-channel pairings and anatomical relationships are combined and guide the selection of areas for treatment. This method is specific: the first approach is to match the corresponding joint and the six-channel pair, and matching both is the primary goal. The following examples show the twelve-joint and six-channel relationships.

1. If there is pain at Kidney 3, treat Heart 7. This treatment is the hand Shaoyin channel treating the foot Shaoyin channel: it is the hand treating the foot.

2. If there is pain at San Jiao 10, treat Gallbladder 34.

3. If there is pain at Spleen 9, treat Lung 5.

4. If there is pain at Spleen 12, treat Lung 1.

If there is pain in between points or areas on the body, find the corresponding area on the contralateral side. For example, if there is pain on the San Jiao channel halfway between San Jiao 10 and San Jiao 4, locate the area halfway between Gallbladder 34 and Gallbladder 40, and then perform the effectiveness test to determine whether to treat it. Use this type of proportional measurement any time points do not anatomically correspond exactly with the twelve-joints relationships. This is anatomical imaging and correspondences.

For all situations, perform the effectiveness test. If the test does not reduce the pain level more than 20 percent, then it's best to treat other locations. In most cases, there will be a substantial decrease in pain; a reduction of 50 percent or more is common.

Application 2

If the effectiveness test does not have a favorable result in application 1, palpate areas around the area first tested and treat the surrounding area if the effectiveness test is positive. The area of treatment can be around the corresponding area; this approach is a type of anatomical imaging, but it is not imaging that includes anatomy *and* acupuncture channels and points.

Application 3
If applications 1 and 2 are not effective, try the same imaged point on same side of the pain. Methods 1 and 2 are contralateral treatments. Always perform the effectiveness test.

Method 2: Yin-Yang channels twelve-joint theory
The Yin-Yang twelve-joint theory utilizes the anatomical relationships between Yin-Yang paired channels. Table 10.2 presents these relationships. This approach is supported by the *Su Wen*, Chapter 5 and *Ling Shu*, Chapter 7.

Table 10.2: Yin-Yang channels twelve-joint theory

Yin-Yang channels	Anatomical relationship	Example
Gallbladder and Liver	Foot to foot	Gallbladder 40 and Liver 4
Bladder and Kidneys	Foot to foot	Bladder 60 and Kidney 3
Heart and Small Intestine	Hand to hand	Heart 7 and Small Intestine 5
Pericardium and San Jiao	Hand to hand	Pericardium 7 and San Jiao 4
Spleen and Stomach	Foot to foot	Spleen 9 and Stomach 36/35
Large Intestine and Lung	Hand to hand	Large Intestine 11 and Lung 5

Anatomically, Yin-Yang paired channels have hand-to-hand and foot-to-foot relationships. An example of this method is left Gallbladder 40 treating pain at right Liver 4, or right Spleen 9 treating pain at left Stomach 36. Apply the effectiveness test before you needle the point.

In the Yin-Yang channels twelve-joint method, as well as for all the methods, test the contralateral area first. If it is not effective, try testing and treating the same side. Be sure to use the effectiveness test every time.

CLINICAL POINT SELECTION

While these pain treatments can be very effective in reducing pain, *they cannot change musculoskeletal structural conditions* (orthopedic or other physical healing modalities may be needed to change structural imbalances). These treatments can be combined with sinew channel treatments, providing an effective local-distal treatment plan.

Chinese medicine is very effective in treating pain. Combining multiple healing modalities generates the best clinical results. In addition to the healing modalities mentioned, bodywork, exercise, medical qi gong and medical yoga (tao yin gentle stretching) have a powerful healing impact as both a preventative measure and a form of treating pain.

CHAPTER 11

Professional Reviews

The Eight Extraordinary Vessels Intersection Points hypothesis and the Source-Luo, Host-Guest point combination

There are two acupuncture theories that have influenced teachers and practitioners and altered the way acupuncture has been practiced since 1295 CE. The two theories are related because they both include the luo points. The first theory begins the process of changing the functions of four luo points and the second theory includes changes to the functions of twelve luo points. The two theories are the *Eight Extraordinary Vessels Intersection Points* (also called the opening, command, confluent points) and the *source-luo points treatment* (also called the host-guest treatment). My review of these theories begins with understanding the luo collaterals in the *Nei Jing*.

Nei Jing luo collaterals theory and applications

The luo mai are primarily presented in Chapter 10 of the *Ling Shu*, "The Main Channels," and they are also presented in many chapters in the *Nei Jing*. The luo mai are also referred to as the luo linking, the connecting vessels or the luo collaterals. The chapter presents specific signs and symptoms in the luo mai, and a treatment method—treat the luo point. This knowledge is the classical clinical application of the luo mai found in Chapter 10 of the *Ling*

123

Shu. The foundation information and functions of the luo mai are given here, along with differences from the main channels.

- The luo mai are located at the superficial region of the body.

- The luo mai flow through the minor joints; they do not flow through the main joints. However, when a pathogen transfers to the main channels, it can flow into the main joints and wherever the main channels flow.

- The luo mai can be visible. When pathogens are lodged in the luo mai, they can be seen. Diagnosis includes visual examination of the luo mai. The main channels cannot be seen.

- The pulse does not detect the luo mai. The pulse does measure the main channels and the internal organs.

- Heat and cold are the main pathogens in the luo mai. Rheumatism occurs when pathogens in the luo mai are not treated effectively.

- The luo mai can have excess and deficiency conditions.

- The luo mai make up a protective channel system that can block and hold pathogens.

- Luo mai treatments release pathogens.

- Pathogens can be transferred from the luo mai to the main channels and the internal organs.

A protective system

From the *Su Wen*, Chapter 56, "Dermatomes of the Channels":

> All disease begins at the skin level. When a pathogen invades the skin it forces the pores to open and pathogens penetrate and lodge in the luo mai. If the pathogen remains it will transfer to the main channels. If the pathogen is not released it will then enter the fu organs.

> The function of the luo mai is to dispel pathogens and promote (allow) the normal flow of the ying and wei qi.
>
> Before a pathogen enters the main channels it can be seen in the luo mai. The luo mai are considered Yang and float to the surface; they can be seen. The main channels are considered Yin because they run relatively deep; they cannot be seen.[1]

From the *Su Wen*, Chapter 58, "Acupuncture Points":

> The collaterals that connect throughout the body act as connectors that can be utilized to release pathogens. They can also supply qi to fight illness. There are 14-main collaterals, and there are numerous tiny collaterals crisscrossing the body, connecting the channels. If a pathogen enters the deep level of the bones, the collaterals are insufficient to treat this condition; the treatment must enter the five main channels of the five zang organs.[2]

The luo mai cannot treat this condition—the luo mai are at the superficial level of the body.

Luo mai pathogens

The pathogenic factors of the luo mai are listed in the *Ling Shu*, Chapter 10, "The Main Channels," and in the *Su Wen*, Chapter 57, "The Channels and Collaterals." These pathogens and conditions are: cold, heat, rheumatism, Qi stagnation and blood stagnation. Temperature, stagnation, deficiency, excess and the changes in the seasons can cause pathology in the luo mai. Heat and cold are the main pathogens in the luo mai. Pathology can show as colors. The changes of the seasons also cause reactions in the luo mai, which are especially susceptible to heat and movement generated by heat. The movement can transfer pathogens within the luo mai and to other areas of the body. The luo mai are also susceptible to

---

[1] Ni, M. (1995) *The Yellow Emperor's Classic of Medicine: A New Translation of Neijing Suwen with Commentary*. Boston, MA: Shambhala.
[2] Ibid.

stagnation, which can lead to fever. The following are the main pathogens in the luo mai.

Heat
Heat and fever are a red color.

When the middle of the Stomach is hot, the luo mai along the border of the fish (thenar eminence) will be red.

Cold
Cold and pain are a blue or green color.

When the middle of the stomach is cold, the fish on the hand (thenar eminence), the base of the thumb's luo mai, will be mostly green-blue.

Cold and heat
When there is both cold and hot qi, there is a red, black and green color.

Cold and heat are red, black and green.

Rheumatism
Rheumatism (bi syndrome) is a black color. It can be an abrupt blackening of the luo mai, and is a sign of prolonged and chronic rheumatism.

Luo mai and colors

- Blue is cold and pain.
- Green is cold and pain.
- Green-blue is cold in the Stomach.
- Red is heat and fever.
- Sudden black is bi syndrome.
- Red, green and black is cold and heat.

Color, location and condition
Thenar eminence

- Blue at the thenar eminence is cold in the Stomach.
- Red at the thenar eminence is heat in the Stomach.
- Black at the thenar eminence is bi syndrome.
- Black, red and blue at the thenar eminence is cold and heat in the Stomach.
- Blue is a short luo mai and is Qi deficiency.
- Blackening is prolonged and chronic rheumatism.
- Green is a short collateral with sparse qi.

Luo mai and the seasons

There are natural colors during the seasons and they are considered normal. The Yin collaterals are the same color as their corresponding organs: the Heart is red, the Spleen is yellow, the Lungs are white, the Kidneys are black and the Liver is green.

The Yang collaterals change color according to seasonal variations:

- During winter and autumn, the cool temperature slows down the flow of the blood and qi. There can be green, blue and black colors.
- During the summer and spring, it is warmer and heat causes a faster flow of the blood and qi. There can be a yellow and red color.

If the body displays all five colors in the collaterals, however, this indicates extreme cold or extreme heat. This acute change is considered pathological.

Luo mai excess and deficiency

The luo mai can suffer from excess and deficiency conditions (shi and xu). The *Ling Shu* presents these two conditions for each of the luo mai. The guidance is that when the 15 luo mai are excess, they are visible, and when they are deficient, they sink. The practitioner should evaluate the luo mai to determine whether the condition is excess (solid) or deficient (hollow).

The following information for excess and deficiency is from the *Ling Shu*, except when there is an asterisk which designates the source as the *Jia Yi Jing*.

Excess and deficiency of the luo collaterals
The arm Taiyin channel (Lungs)

- Excess: The wrist and palm are hot.
- Deficiency: Yawning with the mouth open; frequent urination.

The arm minor Yin channel (Heart)

- Excess: Pressure in the chest.
- Deficiency: Inability to speak.

The hand Jueyin channel (Pericardium)

- Excess: Pain in the Heart.
- Deficiency: Rigidity of the head. (Emotional upset.*)

The arm Taiyang channel (Small Intestine)

- Excess: Loosening of the joints; wasting of the elbows.
- Deficiency: Small swellings. These may be warts and scabs that itch.

The arm Yangming channel (Large Intestine)
- Excess: Toothache; deafness.
- Deficiency: Coldness in the teeth; numbness in the diaphragm.

The arm Shaoyang channel (San Jiao)
- Excess: Dysfunction of the elbow.
- Deficiency: Dysfunction of the elbow.

The leg Taiyang channel (Bladder)
- Excess: Congested nasal passages; pain in the head and neck.
- Deficiency: Bloody nose.

The leg Shaoyang channel (Gallbladder)
- Excess: Deficiencies. Inversion.*
- Deficiency: Paralysis, lameness; inability to rise from a sitting position.

The leg Yangming channel (Stomach)
When there is rebellious qi, there is a numb throat.
- Excess: Madness. Manic. (Mania and withdrawal.*)
- Deficiency: Inflexible foot. The shin withers. Flaccid muscles of the leg.

The leg Taiyin channel (Spleen)
- Excess: Sharp pains in the intestines; abdominal pain.
- Deficiency: Swelling (drum-like) in the intestines; abdominal bloating.

CLINICAL POINT SELECTION

The leg Shaoyin channel (Kidneys)
When there is rebellious and counterflow qi, there is depression and annoyance.

- Excess: Constipation and blockage of urine.
- Deficiency: Pain in the loins. (Low back pain.*)

The leg Jueyin channel (Liver)
When there is rebellious and counterflow qi, there is swelling of the testicles and a hernia.

- Excess: Abnormal erection.
- Deficiency: Severe itching in the groin.

The Ren channel

- Excess: Pain in the skin of the abdomen.
- Deficiency: Itching in the abdomen.

The Du channel

- Excess: Rigidity of the backbone; convulsions.
- Deficiency: Heavy feeling in the head, and shaking at the top of the head.

The great luo of the Spleen

- Excess: Pain throughout the body.
- Deficiency: All the joints are loose. (Slackness in the hundred joints.*)

The luo mai make up a protective channel system; they hold or store pathogens and can be treated to release pathogens from the body. If the pathogens are not correctly treated, they may be transferred to the main channels, and possibly to the internal organs.

They can also transform into bi syndrome. It is essential to treat pathogens before they transfer and cause a more serious condition.

Treating the luo collaterals

Chapter 10 of the *Ling Shu*, "The Main Channels," presents the following guidance:

> The way to treat the luo mai is bloodletting. Even if the pathogens cannot be seen but there are symptoms, treat them to remove the pathogen by bloodletting. If the pathogen is not removed it can transform into rheumatism.[3]

Chapter 10 goes on to state:

> To use acupuncture for these cold and hot diseases, draw much blood from the luo collaterals. Treat once every other day. When this exhaustive bloodletting stops, then harmonize the hollow and the solid.
>
> In extreme cases, to disperse results in depression. When depression is severe, it can result in fainting and in loss of speech; therefore, if there is depression, quickly seat the patient. When there is severe depression do not prick to bleed.[4]

The treatment for the luo mai is *prick to bleed*. There are three suggested places for treatment:

1. The point of separation (the luo point).
2. Where there is a change in color in the luo mai.
3. Where the collaterals are twisted.

Note: "Twisted" can mean that a collateral is "full and firm, protuberant, dark red or purple in color."[5]

There is additional guidance:

---

[3] Wu, J. (2002) *Ling Shu or The Spiritual Pivot*. Hawaii: University of Hawaii Press.
[4] Ibid.
[5] Wang, Z. & Wang, J. (2007) *Ling Shu Acupuncture*. Irvine, CA: Ling Shu Press.

If the pathogen is allowed to become lodged within the luo mai, this gives rise to bi.[6]

In all, there are 15 luo collaterals. When they suffer from a solid disease they become visible. When they suffer from a hollow disease they sink.[7]

Prick to bleed the point of separation (the luo point) is the main method for luo mai treatments. The treatment can be based on visual diagnosis, or on the excess and deficiency conditions of the luo mai. Chapter 10 of the *Ling Shu* presents the excess and deficiency conditions of the luo mai.

It is clear the luo collaterals are used to release pathogens from the superficial level where the luo collaterals are distributed. Bloodletting is the classical treatment that matches the level where the luo collaterals are located. The luo don't treat deep levels of the body and do not treat the internal organs. The information in this chapter is the classical theory and clinical application for the luo collaterals. Any theory that differs from it should include an explanation for the variance using acupuncture theory.

The Eight Extraordinary Vessels Intersection Points hypothesis: A professional review

Dou Hanqing presented the Eight Flowing and Pooling Points in his book *Guide to Acupuncture* in the Yuan dynasty (1295). This presentation of the Eight Flowing and Pooling Points, which are also called the Eight Intersection Points in the original text and commonly referred to as the confluent, master, command and opening points of the Eight Extraordinary Vessels, has three sections. The first section of the text is a chart that is commonly presented in acupuncture texts; the second section is the point location of the

---

6   Wu, J. (2002) *Ling Shu or The Spiritual Pivot*. Hawaii: University of Hawaii Press.
7   Ibid.

points, which is common knowledge in acupuncture texts; and the final section is not presented in common English acupuncture texts but should be, as it may alter the common understanding of the Eight Intersection Points and whether they can actually treat the Eight Extraordinary Vessels.

This chapter includes my analysis (professional review) of the Eight Intersection Points and the Eight Flowing and Pooling Points hypothesis. The goal of this review is to determine if there are theories and clinical applications rooted in classical acupuncture to support the points as being related to the Eight Extraordinary Vessels. This analysis can assist a practitioner in deciding how best to create Eight Extraordinary Vessels treatments.

Four of the Eight Intersection Points are luo points. Understanding the theory and clinical applications of the luo collaterals and the luo points is the base of analysis of the intersection points hypothesis, and any variance from it requires explanation from that theory and clinical application. The luo collaterals and luo points presented at the beginning of this chapter are the source for classical theories and clinical applications for the luo collaterals and luo points.

Dou Hanqing did not present any acupuncture theory supporting the Eight Intersection Points, which is a glaring omission. Since there is no supporting theory in the hypothesis, I include the following acupuncture theories and clinical applications for the reader to review to determine if it might be the basis of the Eight Intersection Points hypothesis.

1. Luo channel trajectory analysis.
2. Eight Extraordinary Channels trajectory analysis.
3. Sinew channel pathology.
4. Luo collateral pathology and clinical applications.
5. Main channel and organ pathology.
6. Eight extraordinary symptoms, conditions and pathology.

CLINICAL POINT SELECTION

The Eight Flowing and Pooling Points (section 1 of *Guide to Acupuncture*)

Table 11.1: The Eight Points of Intersection

Gong Sun (SP 4) communicates with the Chong vessel	They unite in the chest, heart and stomach
Nei Guan (PC 6) communicates with Yin Wei	
Lin Qi (GB 41) communicates with the Dai vessel	They unite in the outer canthus of the eye, (behind the ear, cheek, neck, shoulder, supra-clavicular fossa, chest and diaphragm)
Wai Guan (SJ 5) communicates with Yang Wei	
Hou Xi (SI 3) communicates with the Du vessel	They unite in the inner canthus, neck, (nape, ear, shoulder, arm, small intestine and urinary bladder)
Shen Mai (UB 62) communicates with Yang Qiao	
Lie Que (LU 7) communicates with the Ren vessel	They unite in the lung attachment, throat, chest and diaphragm
Zhao Hai (KI 6) communicates with Yin Qiao	

Table 11.1 above states Gong Sun (Spleen 4) communicates with the Chong vessel. It does not say how Gong Sun (Spleen 4) communicates with the Chong vessel; there is no acupuncture theory to support that claim in the Eight Extraordinary Intersection Points hypothesis.

One analysis a practitioner should perform is a review of the theory, function and clinical applications of the luo collaterals, which includes evaluating the trajectory of the spleen luo collateral, because Spleen 4 is a luo point. I have summarized the foundation information about the luo collaterals and luo points from the classical acupuncture texts: *Nei Jing* (*Inner Classic*) and *Jia Yi Jing* (*Classic of Acupuncture and Moxibustion*) in the introduction to this chapter. The luo collaterals flow at the superficial layer of the body, they can be seen (are visible) and are bled; they do not flow deep into the body, do not influence deep layers of the body

PROFESSIONAL REVIEWS

and cannot treat organs. That trajectory and treatment method is opposite to the Eight Extraordinary Vessels.

The Chong vessel trajectory analysis

The Chong vessel originates in the Lower Jiao and flows to the uterus for females, which is a deep trajectory. The Spleen luo flows at the superficial layer of the body; it is bled to release pathogens in the collateral. The Spleen luo collateral and the Chong vessel flow at opposite levels within the layers of the body. The Spleen luo trajectory does not support that Spleen 4 can treat the Chong vessel. The Spleen 4 "communication" hypothesis does not change the most effective way to treat the Chong channel: treat acupuncture points on the channel. The presentation of the Eight Intersection Points does not state the treatment method to be applied, for example, bloodletting or needling with a standard needle that is used to treat the main channels. The table does not present what exactly the intersection points treat; that is listed in the third section and there is no mention of the Eight Extraordinary Vessels in that section; it only lists that the points treat a variety of conditions.

The intersection table presents that Nei Guan (Pericardium 6) communicates with the Yin Wei vessel. There is no theory presented in the text to support that Nei Guan, Pericardium 6 can treat the Yin Wei vessel. The trajectory of the Yin Wei vessel begins on the lower medial leg at Kidney 9 and flows upward to Spleen 15, Spleen 16 and then Liver 14 and flows to the Heart and to the throat (some sources list Ren 22 and Ren 23). The Pericardium luo collateral begins at Pericardium 6 and flows up the medial arm to the Heart. The Pericardium main channel and luo collateral flow to the Heart and can treat it. Most of the Pericardium luo collateral is on the arm and does not distribute to the lower limb, abdomen and throat. Acupuncture channel trajectory shows the Pericardium luo is not distributed to at least 90 percent of the Yin Wei vessel and does not treat common conditions treated by the Yin Wei vessel; that is presented later in this chapter. From an acupuncture theory viewpoint, one of the channels with points on the Yin Wei vessel would be supported as an intersection point of the Yin Wei vessel.

The intersection table presents that Lie Que (Lung 7) communicates with the Ren vessel. The table and text do not state how that communication occurs. The trajectory of the Lung luo collateral separates from Lung 7 and spreads to the thenar eminence; the trajectory is on the hand only. The Ren vessel starts in the Lower Jiao and flows to the uterus for women. There is no connection from the Lung luo collateral to the Lower Jiao and the uterus. Because the Ren pathway flows to the uterus, it is an important point for treating gynecological conditions. There is no classical theory or channel trajectory that supports treating Lung 7 instead of Ren vessel points for treating the Ren vessel, not even as a supporting acupuncture point in a Ren vessel treatment. Analysis of Lung 7 as the intersection, opening, master or confluent point of the Ren vessel is the most glaring example of a lack of acupuncture theory supporting the Eight Points of Intersection hypothesis.

The intersection points on the Yang and Yin Qiao vessels are on their trajectory and are a logical choice. It is a clinical reality that treating one acupuncture point on a channel is often not enough to effectively treat a condition—it usually takes treating multiple points and this is true for the Eight Extraordinary Vessels too.

The intersection points table presents that Lin Qi (Gallbladder 41) communications with the Dai vessel. The *Nei Jing* Dai vessel contains three Gallbladder points: 26, 27, 28. Since Gallbladder 41 is on the same channel as the Dai vessel points, there is some trajectory support. The clinical treatment question is whether Gallbladder 41 can treat the Dai vessel alone or whether it is more effective to treat the Dai vessel points and maybe include Gallbladder 41 as support. The *Ling Shu*, Chapter 1 provides fundamental treatment guidance for any condition: treat the channel directly, that is, Gallbladder 26, 27 and 28.

Performing the same analysis on the Du and Yang Wei vessels reveals that there is no acupuncture channel theory supporting them as intersection points with their "related" Eight Extraordinary Vessel, and most importantly, that the practitioner would not use those points instead of points on the Extraordinary Vessels.

Section 2 of the Eight Intersection Points of the Eight Extraordinary Vessels hypothesis presents the point location of the Eight Intersection Points. No analysis is necessary.

The Eight Points and treatment of symptoms (section 3 *of Guide to Acupuncture*)

This section of Dou Hanqing's presentation includes the Eight Intersection Points and the conditions they treat. It is in this section that we seek to understand if there is any acupuncture theory to support the conditions being treated and, most importantly, do they relate to the corresponding Eight Extraordinary Vessel? In an effort to bring clarity to the evaluation I have listed what the points treat from classical and traditional conditions based on acupuncture channel theory, including the channel system—sinew channels, luo collaterals, main channels and the Eight Extraordinary Vessels—as the basis of comparison.

The purpose of this review is to determine if there are classical and traditional acupuncture theories to support the Eight Intersection Points of the Eight Extraordinary Points. I have selected three points: Gong Sun (Spleen 4), Lie Que (Lung 7) and Nei Guan (Pericardium 6) for a detailed analysis that will help to answer the question of whether there is acupuncture theory to support the Eight Intersection Points hypothesis.

> Gong Sun (Spleen 4), bilateral point, governs the treatment of twenty-seven symptoms.
>
> Nine types of angina, phlegm, distension and pain of the abdomen and umbilicus, pain in the hypochondriac region, coma after women gave birth, difficult labor, blockage of the trachea, blockage of the esophagus, diarrhea, pain caused by sexual disease, dysentery, febrile disease, phlegm caused by drinking wine, vomiting, and distention of the abdomen and hypochondriac region, blood

stool, collapse of rectum pain due to stagnation of food, anorexia in children, occipital pain in children, abdominal pain due to diarrhea, needling pain in the chest, malaria.[8]

Gong Sun (Spleen 4) is indicated for all the above disease symptoms. First apply treatment at Gong Sun, then treat Nei Gong (Pericardium 6).

Author's note: The text presents that Spleen 4 can treat the conditions listed above; it does not say that those conditions are related to the Chong channel. The text does not list the source for the 27 symptoms that Spleen 4 treats. The text does not say if the conditions are excess or deficient and does not indicate whether to reinforce or reduce Spleen 4.

In an attempt to identify any source for the conditions that Spleen 4 can treat according to Dou Hanqing's presentation I have listed conditions treated from each of the Spleen channel systems.

Classical and traditional channels and luo point functions
Sinew channel
Pulling/stiffness of the big toe, pain medial malleolus, spasm/pain medial aspect leg, spasm/pulling pain/cold/twisting sensation of the external genitalia, pain around umbilicus, pulling pain intercostal region.

Spleen luo collateral
Luo collaterals:

- Full/excess: Colic pain of stomach/intestines.

- Empty/deficiency: Abdominal distention, ascites, childhood nutritional impairment, flatulence.

Great luo collateral of Spleen:

---

8   Wang, Z. & Wang, J. (2007) *Ling Shu Acupuncture.* Irvine, CA: Ling Shu Press.

- Full/excess: Whole body pain, multiple site arthritis, bi syndrome.
- Empty/Deficiency: Muscular atrophy/flaccidity, joint weakness, whole body weakness.

Primary channel
Heavy sensation head/body, facial puffiness, swelling legs/feet/joints, loss of capability to roll or extend tongue, tongue stiffness, impaired speech, pain/cold/hot along medial thigh/knee/foot/toe, wei syndrome, pain in cheek/mandible.

Organ disorder
Epigastric pain, loose stools, diarrhea, borborygmus, vomiting, nausea, abdominal fullness/distention, reduced appetite, jaundice, lassitude, listlessness, abdominal Qi masses, leukorrhea, excess phlegm fluid, difficult urination, edema.

Chong mai
Sea of Blood, sea of the twelve primary channels.

Gynecological disorders, sexual disorders, impotence, spasm and pain in the abdomen, irregular menses, infertility, asthmatic breathing, dyspnea, colic, running piglet, counterflow qi, atrophy disorders of the leg.

Channel trajectory analysis
The Chong Mai's main trajectory begins in the Lower Jiao (Kidneys) and flows to the uterus and up the center line.

Spleen luo collateral begins at Spleen 4 and does not flow to the Kidneys/Jing, uterus or the center line.

	Spleen luo collateral	Chong vessel
Location	Superficial	Deep
Treatment	Bleed	Needle

CLINICAL POINT SELECTION

Lie Que (Lung 7), bilateral point, governs the treatment of thirty-one symptoms.

Cold pain and diarrhea, postpartum blood lump with pain or retention of normal postpartum discharge (lochia), swollen and painful throat (pharyngitis, tonsillitis), fetus dies and will not deliver, teeth sullen and painful, small intestine spasm pain (such as a hernia that protrudes on the abdomen), stagnation on one side of the abdomen with pain, vomiting saliva with pus and blood, coughing with cold mucous, pulling qi pain in the muscles below the ribs (or severe tension between the scapulae or severe tension at the side of the navel caused by cold wind invading the uterus, stagnant food and digestive problems, sharp pain in the umbilicus and abdomen, pain of the heart and abdomen, borborygmus and diarrhea, itchy, painful, bleeding hemorrhoids, heart pain, lumbar pain following labor, madness after labor, inability to speak after labor, inability to digest rice and grains, stagnation of one side of the abdomen caused by alcohol, the food won't pass; swelling-abscess on the sides of the breast (mastitis), stagnant blood lump in women, chronic external febrile disease, ceaseless vomiting, blood in the urine, inability to pass urine, constipation, blood in the feces, painful disease of the stomach/intestine, any lump.[9]

Lie Que (Lung 7) is indicated for all the above disease symptoms. First apply treatment at Lie Que, then apply treatment at Zhao Hai (Kidney 6).

Author's note: The text presents that Lung 7 can treat the conditions listed, but it does not say that those conditions are related to the Ren channel. The text does not list the source for the 31 symptoms that Lung 7 treats. The text does not indicate whether the conditions are excess or deficient and does not say whether to reinforce or reduce Lung 7.

---

9   Matsumoto, K. & Birch, S. (1986) *Extraordinary Vessels*. Brookline, MA: Paradigm Publications.

Classical and traditional channels and luo point functions
Lung luo collateral

- Full/excess: Heat in the wrist and palm.
- Empty/deficiency: Yawning and frequent urination.

Sinew channel
Conditions include cramping of the muscles along their pathways. Extreme pain in the cardiac orifice that may cause panting. Spasms in the ribs may cause the spitting of blood.

Main channel
Conditions include coughing, rebellious qi, panting and thirst, an anxious Heart, a congested chest, pain and spasms in the shoulder bone and the medial anterior surface of the upper arm, and heat in the center of the palm. When the Qi is full and there is excess, it results in the shoulder and back being painful from wind and cold. There will be sweating from the attacking wind. Urination is frequent but scanty. When Qi is empty, it results in the shoulder and back being painful from cold. Sparse Qi is in accord with an insufficiency of breathing. There will be change in the color of urine.

Lung organ
Cough, asthma, shortness of breath, sputum, hemoptysis, weak voice, fatigue, frequent colds, chest pain with a stifling sensation, palpitations, restlessness, smooth frequent urination, incontinence, edema, abdominal fullness/distension, loose stools, diarrhea, constipation, and burning pain in the epigastrium or behind the sternum.

Ren vessel
Sea of Yin channels. Receive and bear the Qi of Yin channels.

Leucorrhoea, irregular menses, colic, infertility, hernia,

nocturnal emission, enuresis, retention of urine, pain in epigastric region and lower abdomen, pain in genital region.

Channel trajectory analysis
Ren vessel's main trajectory begins deep in the Lower Jiao at the Kidneys and flows to the uterus and then up the center line of the body.
Lung luo collateral begins on the hand and flows to the thenar eminence. It is on the hand only.

	Lung luo collateral	Ren vessel
Location	Superficial	Deep
Treatment	Bleed	Needle

Nei Guan (Pericardium 6), bilateral point, governs the treatment of twenty-five symptoms.

Fullness condition with discomfort on the inside, stagnation and fullness in the heart and chest, irregular vomiting, feeling of fullness in the chest caused by a deficient/damp spleen with mucous, abdominal pain, water diarrhea or frequent stools, alcohol mucous, inability to transform rice and grains, lump in the inguinal crease, anal prolapse in children, pain in the sides of the rib cage, blood stabbing pain in women, "two diaphragm" feeling of fullness and distension around the diaphragm, diaphragm and food stagnation, heart and rib cage swollen and painful, intestinal wind and bleeding from the anus, anus pain following a bout of diarrhea, stagnant food in the diaphragm.[10]

Nei Guan (Pericardium 6) is indicated for all the above disease symptoms.

Author's note: The text presents that Pericardium 6 can treat the conditions listed, but it does not say those conditions are related

---

10 Matsumoto, K. & Birch, S. (1986) *Extraordinary Vessels*. Brookline, MA: Paradigm Publications.

to the Yin Wei channel. The text does not list the source for the 25 symptoms that Pericardium 6 treats. The text does not indicate whether the conditions are excess or deficient and does not say whether to reinforce or reduce the Pericardium 6.

The Eight Extraordinary Vessels have systemic functions. The Yin Wei vessel is treated when all Yin and Yang is not linked (one is upset and loses one's mind). There is no mention of this systemic function. The conditions appear to be related to the main channel and the luo collateral trajectories as they flow to the Heart.

Classical and traditional channels and luo point functions
Luo collaterals

- Full/excess: Heart pain, chest pain, angina.
- Empty/deficiency: Vexation in the Heart, restlessness, irritability, stiffness of head.

Sinew channel
Stiffness/pulling/spasm/pain along channel, chest pain, stuffiness of chest, mass below right hypochondrium which may be a tumor/lung abscess/tuberculosis/pleurisy, may have cough, harsh/rapid/painful breathing, hemoptysis, vomiting.

Primary channel
Pain/stiffness neck/hands/feet, swelling axillary region, inability to extend/flex elbow, forearm spasms, hot palms, fullness chest/hypochondriac region.

Organ disorder
Palpitations, cardiac pain, restlessness, stuffiness in chest, high lipid levels, delirium, syncope, incessant laughing, depression, anxiety, manic depression.

Yin Wei vessel
Links or connects all Yin channels. Dominates the interior of body. Interior syndromes such as heart pain, chest pain, cardiac pain and stomachache, digestion, nausea, vomiting, insomnia, emotional disturbance, Shen disturbance, fullness and pain of the lateral costal region, mental disorders.

Channel trajectory analysis
Yin Wei vessel is primarily on the leg and abdomen and does not flow on the arm. Pericardium luo is primarily on the arm.

	Pericardium luo collateral	Yin Wei vessel
Location	Superficial	Deep
Treatment	Bleed	Needle

Summary

On reviewing the classical theories and clinical applications of the early texts of acupuncture it is clear that the Intersection Points of the Eight Extraordinary Vessels hypothesis is not supported by acupuncture theory. I suggest the reader refer to acupuncture books and review the pathways of the channel system to confirm the lack of support for Intersection Points in any channel theory.

The Eight Intersection Points theory does not explain why the eight points were selected or why a particular point was selected among the other acupuncture points on its channel. The hypothesis clearly states that each intersection point treats specific conditions; it does not state they treat the Eight Extraordinary Vessels. It seems that other practitioners make that leap to treating the Eight Extraordinary Vessels and its pathology and functions. That leap should be fully evaluated to determine whether it leads to an effective treatment.

It is very interesting that the legendary Li Shizhen did not include the Eight Intersection Points in his book *An Exposition of the Eight Extraordinary Vessels: Acupuncture, Alchemy and Herbal*

Medicine. It seems evident from reading his book that he did not see any acupuncture theory to support the intersection points and therefore omitted them. I agree with that omission. One of the main problems seen in teachings and clinical practice in the acupuncture profession is how this hypothesis changes the way practitioners create Eight Extraordinary Vessels treatments. It is common for practitioners to treat only the intersection point (opening, command, master) and not to treat points on the Eight Extraordinary Vessels, which is a contradiction of the *Ling Shu*'s principle number one for creating acupuncture treatments: *identify the imbalanced channel and treat it at those locations*. Treatment of the Eight Extraordinary Vessels requires treating them directly, as the primary treatment. Analysis of the intersection point hypothesis provides the practitioner with the knowledge to create acupuncture treatments that are customized for each patient rather than treating points and channels unrelated to the Eight Extraordinary Vessels.

I hope this review motivates analysis and discussion on how to most effectively treat the Eight Extraordinary Vessels.

Source-Luo points treatment (also called the host-guest treatment): A professional review

Changes to the classical luo collaterals theory and clinical applications

The structure, function and treatments for the luo mai have changed from the time of the *Su Wen* and the *Ling Shu*. I presented *Nei Jing Su Wen* and *Ling Shu* luo collaterals theories and applications in the introduction to this chapter. A series of changes in the theory and function of the luo collaterals and luo points began around 1295 CE and continued to the mid-1950s.

Dou Hanqing created the first change in luo points theory and functions when he presented his hypothesis of the Eight Intersection Points (command, opening, confluent, master points) for the

Eight Extraordinary Vessels in 1295 CE. Four of the intersection points are luo points. The functions of those luo points would expand from the *Ling Shu*, *Su Wen* and other early acupuncture classics to include treating their associated Eight Extraordinary Vessels and the indications listed in Dou Hanqing's *Guide to Acupuncture*.

The second change occurred in *The Great Compendium of Acupuncture and Moxibustion (Zhen Jiu Da Cheng)*, written by Yang Jizhou in the Ming dynasty. Yang presented the source-luo, host-guest method, where the source and luo points treat imbalances of each channel system.

The third change occurred with George Soulié De Morant, the French practitioner, writer and teacher. He devised the transverse luo channel theory to explain how Yang's host-guest method worked, and promoted using only the luo point and not the source-luo point combination in treatment.

The fourth change occurred with the French physician Dr. Albert Chamfrault and the influential Vietnamese translator, teacher and practitioner Dr. Nguyen Van Nghi, who both further developed the transverse luo channel theory and included the source-luo points combination in treatment.

Each of the theories, interpretations, assumptions and applications will be evaluated to gain a deeper understanding of them, which will be a guide in determining if there is any relationship to the teachings from the Han dynasty classics—*Nei Jing Su Wen* and *Ling Shu*.

The first change in the luo collaterals theory and clinical application

Dou Hanqing is a famous practitioner and writer of Chinese acupuncture and his book, *The Guide of Acupuncture*, was published around 1295 CE. Dou Hanqing is the person we can trace to the initial presentation of the Eight Intersection Points (command, opening, confluent, master points) of the Eight Extraordinary Vessels. The intersection points' category and function were not in any known texts before his text. He left no meaningful theory about how they work or why each point was selected, and for that reason some practitioners do not use the points as intersection (opening) points of the Eight Extraordinary Vessels—classical practitioners treat points on the Eight Extraordinary Vessels pathways. See my professional review of the Eight Intersection Points of the Eight Extraordinary Vessels earlier in this chapter for a detailed analysis of that theory. Four luo points were selected as intersection points (opening, command, master or confluent points): Lie Que (Lung 7) for the Ren vessel, Wai Guan (San Jiao 5) for the Yang Wei vessel, Nei Guan (Pericardium 6) for the Yin Wei vessel, and Gong Sun (Spleen 4) for the Chong vessel. Creating this new point category and assigning this function to the four luo points created new conditions those luo points could treat. That new function radically changed the function of those luo points—which now treat the Eight Extraordinary Vessels according to the new theory.

The second change in the luo collaterals theory and clinical application

The second change in luo point functions is found in the *Great Compendium* by Jizhou Yang in the Ming dynasty; the new use of the luo points is the source-luo point combination, which is called the host-guest treatment (there are other versions of the host-guest method). To begin evaluating the host-guest/source-luo point combination it is necessary to understand *Ling Shu*, Chapter 9, "Beginnings and Ends," which presents a diagnostic and treatment method. The chapter introduces the Renying-Cunkou pulse to identify the imbalanced channel which is to be the focus of treatment. The plan is to treat the imbalanced channel and its Yin-Yang paired channel and to balance them—since they connect to each other they influence each other. The needling technique to balance the channels is to reinforce or reduce the imbalanced channel and apply the opposite needling technique on the paired channel. For example, if the foot Taiyin, the Spleen channel is deficient, reinforce the Spleen's channel points to treat the condition

CLINICAL POINT SELECTION

and then reduce the foot Yangming, the Stomach channel's point. This is treating Yin-Yang paired main channels and applying a combination of reinforcing and reducing needling techniques to balance the channels. This is a host-guest treatment comprising Yin-Yang channel pairs, it's not a fixed source-luo points treatment on Yin-Yang paired channels. The guidance is for the practitioner to select the points or areas that treat the condition of the patient, it is not selecting a fixed pair of points for all conditions.

The Renying-Cunkou pulse diagnosis and treatment method includes treating the main channel points or palpating the main channels for stagnations, blockages and knots which are then treated (that approach is found in the *Ling Shu*, Chapter 64, "Yin and Yang and the Twenty-Five Types of Men." The Renying-Cunkuo treatment occurs on the main channels; it is not a luo collaterals treatment. The Renying-Cunkou diagnosis and treatment method contains the fundamental principles of acupuncture found in the *Ling Shu*, Chapter 3, which involves identifying the imbalanced channel and treating it at those locations, and *Ling Shu*, Chapter 1—which involves applying a reinforcing or reducing method.

The Great Compendium of Acupuncture and Moxibustion (*Zhen Jiu Da Cheng*) is a collection of information from the Han to the Ming dynasties, completed in 1601 CE by Jizhou Yang. The *Da Cheng* is a Ming dynasty classic medical text. It includes information from the classics and from unknown sources, as well as his family traditions and his own insights. That classic book is the source of the host-guest, source-luo point combination. Jizhou Yang lists each of the source and luo points for the Yin-Yang paired channels, and the symptoms and conditions that each acupuncture point/channel treats. Classically, when referring to the luo mai, one would use the name luo mai (luo collaterals) to distinguish them from other channel systems, for instance, *the lung sinew channel, the lung divergent channel, the lung main channel* and *the lung luo collateral*. Jizhou Yang does not list the source-luo point combination as a luo mai treatment. He lists them according to

PROFESSIONAL REVIEWS

their organ name, which is a way to reference the main channels. Because the main channels connect to the internal organs, treating the main channels can influence the organs. The way he names this combination is important—it is logical to perceive that he is saying this treatment is treating the main channels and the organs. This approach is not a luo mai treatment. It seems the luo point is supporting the treatment, but it is not explained how.

Jizhou Yang does not cite any sources for the source-luo point combination, in fact they are not found in any classic texts before the *Da Cheng*. The sequence of changing the function of the luo points begins with Dou Hanqing and continues with Jizhou Yang. The shift from treating luo mai symptoms and conditions to treating the Eight Extraordinary Vessels, the main channels and the internal organs is found with Dou Hangqing and Jizou Yang. Most interestingly, there is no theory to support their theories and applications. It was later practitioners and writers that attempted to explain the reasoning for the new functions of the luo mai.

Jizhou Yang offers little guidance about the clinical method for applying a source-luo combination. He does not state whether to reinforce or reduce the points, and that varies from the *Ling Shu*, Chapter 9, which states to reinforce the deficient channel and reduce its Yin-Yang paired channel. Jizhou Yang offers no theory to explain how this point combination works. Morant, Chamfrault and Van Nghi later offered theories about how this combination works, and this changed the theory and function of the luo mai in Europe and later around parts of the world.

The *Da Cheng* includes symptoms for the source-luo points that indicate when to use them for treatment. Jizhou Yang defines the method as the "host-guest" (it is one of a variety of acupuncture combinations that are guest-host combinations). The list of conditions the point combination can treat expands beyond the luo collaterals indications listed in the *Ling Shu*. It is a radical shift in the function of the luo points. Jizhou Yang does not distinguish what the luo points treat from what the source points treat. And he does not describe how they support each other or how they function together.

Jizhou Yang lists some symptoms from the luo mai found in Chapter 10 of the *Ling Shu*. He also adds symptoms from the main channels from the same chapter, as well as symptoms of the internal organs. Unlike the *Ling Shu*, which lists symptoms for excess and deficient conditions of the luo collaterals, Yang does not list conditions in that way. He makes a major shift and variance from the *Ling Shu* in the functions of the luo points. The following is an example of Jizhou Yang's presentation of the source-luo point combination from the *Da Cheng*:

> The twelve channels treat patterns using host-guest, source-luo points. Lung as the host, large intestine as the guest: Taiyin has copious qi and scant blood; qi distention of the heart and chest, feverish palms. No one can avoid panting and cough, pain in the supraclavicular fossa; swollen or dry throat, body sweating more and more. Pain in the medial anterior shoulder and the two breasts; phlegm binding the diagram, qi is lacking.
>
> What points should we seek for disease which is engendered? Speak with a gentlemen about Tai Yuan (Lung 9) and Pi Lian (Large Intestine 6).[11]

Now let's compare those functions to the luo collaterals functions found in the *Ling Shu*. The hand Taiyin collateral treats heat, cold and rheumatism in the collateral.

- Excess: Toothache, deafness.
- Deficiency: Teeth sensitive to cold, bi conditions.

The differences in functions are the inclusion of the hand Taiyin main channel (Lung channel) and some Lung organ functions. Jizhou Yang offers no acupuncture theory as to how the luo point can treat all the conditions.

---

11   Wilcox, L. (2010) *The Great Compendium of Acupuncture and Moxibustion.* Volume V. Portland, OR: The Chinese Medicine Database.

Wide and narrow theory and applications

A common approach in acupuncture point selection is "wide and narrow." A wide view of host-guest is treating Yin-Yang paired channels—that approach is a channel relationship. That channel relationship is found in the *Ling Shu*, Chapter 9, "From Beginning to End." In that chapter, the guidance is to pick three points: two points on one channel and one point on the Yin-Yang paired channel. The guidance does not tell the practitioner which points to treat, but assumes the practitioner will know which points and the areas of channels to treat—that guidance is a wide approach. Jizhou Yang's host-guest method constitutes a narrow view, as it states the points to treat for every treatment—the source and luo points. There is no variation or customization of point selection for each patient's unique condition in Yang's host-guest method.

The third change in the luo collaterals theory and clinical application

George Soulié De Morant was a pioneer in bringing acupuncture from China to France, he promoted the host-guest, source-luo point combination treatment to the Western community. His book, *Chinese Acupuncture*, may have been the first major book on Chinese medicine in France. Morant studied medicine in China for a short period of time. He references two important Ming dynasty books as the reference for his luo mai theory and application. The first text is *The Great Compendium of Acupuncture and Moxibustion* (*Zhen Jiu Da Cheng*) by Jizhou Yang, and the second source is the *Yixue Rumen* (*Introduction to Medicine*) by Li Can.

Morant's theory and method

Morant alters the full method of the host-guest treatment found in the *Ling Shu* Chapter 9 and in Yang's source-luo presentation. He promotes the use of only the luo point to treat any condition of the main channels and the internal organs. He varies from the *Da Cheng* in that his first treatment approach is to use only the luo point of the deficient channel/organ, for example he believed by reinforcing the Kidneys, the Bladder would automatically be reduced and a balance would occur between both channels and organs.

While Jizhou Yang does not present a theory for how the source-luo point combination worked, Morant does. His theory started a stream of theories and clinical practices that brought about a major change in how the luo mai were viewed and applied in clinical practice. Morant proposes that the luo mai have transverse channels where Qi and blood can be transferred between the Yin-Yang paired luo collateral and main channel and the internal organs. For example, when reinforcing Liver 5, the Liver luo point, the Gallbladder main channel and organ will be reduced, balancing both channels. In this theory, treating Liver 5 causes a reaction that both brings Qi into the Liver to supplement it, and reduces or pulls away imbalances in the Gallbladder, creating a balance between both channels and organs. The balance occurs by way of the transverse luo channel.

Morant provides interpretations of the entire channel system that differ from classical Chinese medical sources. He calls the luo collaterals the secondary channels. In Chapter V of his book, "The Fifteen Secondary Vessels," he states the following:

> These luo or secondary vessels and their point of passage are an important element in the circulation of energy. They are branches that connect the paired channels; ie, send the energy from the yin to its coupled yang meridian and from the yang meridian to its coupled yin meridian.[12]

Morant states that if a meridian is empty and its coupled meridian is full, tonification of the point of passage (luo point) of the empty meridian is enough to replenish it, while at the same time the coupled meridian in excess will become normal. Morant uses the luo point to transport Qi and blood between Yin-Yang main channels. This is a new way to use the luo collaterals in acupuncture.

---

12   Morant, G.S. de (1972 French edition, 1994 English edition) *Chinese Acupuncture*. Chapter V. Brookline, MA: Paradigm Publications.

This application ignores two fundamental aspects of the luo mai: the releasing pathogenic factors in the luo mai, and that the luo mai are distributed on the superficial areas of the body, they do not flow deep into the body and do not influence the organs. In Morant's theory, the practitioner must be cautious not to transfer pathogenic factors from the luo point/luo collateral to the main channel and to the internal organs; he does not explain how to avoid this. Morant does not explain the variance from the fundamental function of the luo mai.

Chapter 9 of the *Ling Shu* clearly presents a method to treat imbalances of the main channels and the internal organs. The method is to select the Yin-Yang main channel pairs to balance and treat the condition. For example, if the Spleen channel or organ is deficient, include the Stomach primary channel points along with the Spleen primary channel points to treat the condition. *The main channels are a direct way to influence their channels and the internal organs because the main channel's internal pathways connect to their own organ and their Yin-Yang paired channel's organ; that is why they are Yin-Yang pairs—without a connection there can't be an influence.* The main channel's acupuncture point categories are on the main channels. Morant selects a luo point, which influences the luo collaterals and pathogens in it to treat the main channels and the internal organs. This theory and application contradict the foundation theory and application in the classics of acupuncture. The method has risks, as it can transfer pathogens deeper within the body. The classics offer ways to treat the main channels and the internal organs. One such way is treating the transporting points, which is a main point category in every system of classical and traditional acupuncture; additionally, treating a source point is also a way to treat any condition on a main channel and with an organ. Luo points do not treat the main channels and internal organs.

The fourth change in the luo collaterals theory and clinical application

Dr. Nguyen Van Nghi (NVN) was born in Vietnam and is an important scholar, writer, teacher and practitioner of modern times. Many of his theories and applications are sources used by modern teachers from Europe and the United States. NVN was an allopathic physician. He studied Chinese medicine after practicing Western medicine; he would go on to dedicate his life to Chinese medicine.

Dr. Nguyen Van Nghi moved to France and eventually collaborated with French practitioners. One significant collaboration was with Dr. Albert Chamfrault, who carried on the tradition of Morant's teachings. Through this collaboration it appears that Van Nghi integrated some of the language Morant used into his explanation of Chinese acupuncture. Chamfrault and NVN expand on Morant's theory of transverse luo collaterals and the transfer of Qi by using the source-luo point combination. NVN promotes combining the source and the luo point to transfer Qi between Yin-Yang channels; the transfer is through the transverse luo collaterals. However, as stated before, there is no mention of transverse luo collaterals in any classic or traditional Chinese medical text.

The transverse luo channel theory ignores one main aspect of the luo mai: pathogens can transfer from the luo mai to the main channels and the internal organs. The *Su Wen*, Chapter 63, "Acupuncturing the Superficial Luo," states:

> In general, when a pathogen invades the body, it first enters the skin level. If it lingers or is not expelled, it will travel into the micro luo. If it still is not expelled, it then travels to the regular luo channels. From here it proceeds to the main channels, connecting to the five zang organs, and finally to the intestines and stomach. At this stage, everything may be affected.[13]

---

13 Ni, M. (1995) *The Yellow Emperor's Classic of Medicine: A New Translation of Neijing Suwen with Commentary.* Boston, MA: Shambhala.

That *Su Wen* passage describes the transfer of pathogens from the luo mai to the main channels, the internal organs and potentially everywhere in the body.

The transfer of Qi and blood in the way NVN proposes is an entirely new idea to Chinese acupuncture. The theory references Jizhou Yang's *Great Compendium* (*Da Cheng*), which was then altered by Morant. NVN provides his own theory which is not found in any of the earlier Chinese medical classics, to support his method. NVN differs from Morant in that he suggests to always apply the source-luo point combination. *He states that the transverse channel flows from the luo point to the source point.*

Both Morant and NVN suggest that the widest range of conditions can be treated in their hypothesis: any condition of the Yin-Yang paired channels' channel system (sinew, luo and main channels). The creation of the transverse luo theory is an attempt to explain how the source-luo point combination functions.

NVN presents the idea that there are two collaterals within the luo mai. The first is the collateral found in the *Ling Shu*, which he labels the *longitudinal luo collateral*. He also presents pathways from the luo point (which he calls a reunion point) to the paired Yin-Yang channel. Those pathways are labeled the *transverse luo collaterals*. This explanation can be viewed as formulating a theory to support Morant's transfer of Qi and blood theory. Eventually, the theory was applied to the *Da Cheng*'s source-luo point combination, meaning that the transverse luo mai flows from a luo point to its paired channel's source point. And the transfer of Qi and blood is between those two points by way of the transverse luo pathway. This theory is used to support the source-luo point treatment.

Analysis of the location of the transverse luo

The *Ling Shu*, Chapter 10, "The Main Channels," presents the pathways of the main channels. At each luo point there is a vague description of a branch that flows from that point to its Yin-Yang paired channel. Below are three translations of the descriptions of this branch; the third is from NVN, followed by his comment.

CLINICAL POINT SELECTION

Translation 1

From the Arm Major Yin Channel, the separation of the luo linking channel is at the point called Crack of Lightning. This linking channel starts in the space on top of the wrist, goes along with the Major Yin.

Treat by going to one and one-half cun beyond the wrist (at Lung 7). At this point, a separate branch travels to the Bright Yang.[14]

Author's note:

- Arm Major Yin Channel is the Lungs.
- Crack of Lighting is Lie Que (Lung 7).
- Bright Yang is the Large Intestine.

Translation 2

The [vessel] diverging from the hand major yin [conduit] is called [after the opening where it diverges from the [conduit] *lie que*. It originates from the space above the wrist and extends along the major yin conduits. It enters straight into the palm, where it dissipates and enters the borderline of the ball of the hand.

The [disease] is to be removed in a distance of one and a half inches from the wrist. *[Another] course diverges from the yang brilliance [conduit]*.[15]

Author's note:

- Yang brilliance is Yangming, the Large Intestine.

---

14 Wu, J. (2002) *Ling Shu or The Spiritual Pivot*. Hawaii: University of Hawaii Press.
15 Unschuld, P. (2016) *Huang Di Nei Jing Ling Shu: The Ancient Classic on Needle Therapy*. University of California Press.

Translation 3 (from NVN)

> The luobie (longitudinal or distinct luo) of the Hand Taiyin (Lung) is called Lieque (Lung 7). It starts above the wrist, runs alongside the principal route (channel) of the taiyin (Lung), penetrates into the palm of the hand and branches to the thenar eminence.
>
> It is advised to needle the point Lieque (Lung 7), located 1 1/2 cun above the wrist. *From this point, another vessel (transversal luo or luo yin) also leaves that goes toward the Hand Yangming (Large Intestine).*[16]

From NVN:

> Chamfrault and ourselves have given the name "transversal luo" to all the luo-yin leaving from the luo point of the yin channel toward a yang channel, and vice versa.[17]

Luo collaterals presented in the *Nei Jing* and traditional acupuncture books are what NVN calls the longitudinal luo, and the branch from the luo collateral to its Yin-Yang paired channel is what NVN calls the transverse luo channel. That transverse luo is the basis of his hypothesis—that the transverse luo is what connects *the source and luo points* on Yin-Yang paired channels. The *Ling Shu* does not state that the pathway flows from the luo collateral to the source point on the Yin-Yang paired channel; it states that it flows to the Yin-Yang channel. Morant, Chamfrault and NVN connect that statement to Jizhou Yang's source-luo point treatment. Yang does not offer that theory.

Analysis of the transverse luo

Morant, Chamfrault and NVN hypothesized that the way the source-luo point combination works is by way of a *transverse luo channel* that connects the luo point to its Yin-Yang paired channel at the source point. Morant says the branch off the luo points

---

16 Nghi, N.V., Tran, D. and Nguyen, C. (2002) *Huang Di Nei Jing Ling Shu*. Sugar Grove, NC: Jung Tao School of Classic Chinese Medicine.
17 Ibid.

in the *Ling Shu* references presented above is the transverse luo channel. He is hypothesizing that the branch flows from the luo point, which is at the superficial layer of the body, to the source point on the main channel, and the main channel's internal pathway that flows deep and connects to organs. He suggests that the luo point and its traverse channel connect the exterior to the interior via a connection to the Yin-Yang paired channel's source point.

A common modern method is to tonify the source point on the deficient channel and reduce its Yin-Yang paired channel's luo point, or the opposite needling technique for an excess. The theory is that the needling technique of reinforcing and reducing on the source and luo points on Yin-Yang paired channels creates a push and pull action where two channels work as one to achieve the treatment objective. Applying the reinforcing and reducing needling technique in the treatment is following the guidance in Chapter 9 of the *Ling Shu*.

Variance and conflict between the transverse luo channel hypothesis and classical traditional acupuncture theory

NVN does not discuss the functions of the luo collaterals presented in classical and traditional books prior to Yang's *Great Compendium*. He does not reconcile the conflicts in his theory with the functions of the luo collaterals. There are two aspects of the classical and traditional functions of the luo collaterals that are in direct conflict with Morant's teachings and one main assumption in the hypothesis. The first conflict is that the luo collaterals are located at the superficial area of the body; they do not flow internally to the organs and cannot treat the internal organs. The second is the luo collaterals are a buffer to hold pathogens to prevent them from flowing into the channels and organs. The luo collaterals are bled to release pathogens; they are not needled. The treatment is to release pathogens in the collaterals, preventing them from moving deeper into the body.

Morant does not discuss the reasoning or logic in the change in functions of the luo collaterals.

The main assumption of the transverse luo hypothesis is about the branch off the luo collateral, which is presented below and is also mentioned above:

> Treat by going to one and one-half cun beyond the wrist (at Lung 7). *At this point, a separate branch travels to the Bright Yang.*[18]

The separate branch is where they make an assumption; they believe it connects from the luo collateral to the main channel and the source point of the Yin-Yang paired channel system. The classics do not use precise language regarding the location it travels or flows, but the basic qualities of the luo collaterals provide the foundation for analysis. Since the luo collaterals are located at the superficial area of the body and are bled to release pathogens, it is strongly supported that the separate branch connects to the bright Yang luo collateral (Large Intestine luo collateral), and the Yin-Yang paired luo collaterals would establish a superficial network of luo collaterals. Wang and Wang in their book *Ling Shu Acupuncture* address this issue:

> The collateral of the Hand Taiyin Meridian is what is known as the Collateral of the Hand Taiyin today. Regardless of how large collaterals are, they flow directly off the regular Meridians. Therefore, *Ling Shu* refers to them as the superficial branches of the Meridians.
>
> The Collateral of the Hand-Taiyin connects with the Hand-Taiyin and Hand-Yangming meridian. The Collateral of the Hand-Yangming does the same. *These two collaterals establish the external relationship between the Hand-Taiyin and Hand-Yangming.*[19]

Wang and Wang clearly state where the separate branch connects—*luo collateral to luo collateral.* The collaterals establish the

---

18 Wu, J. (2002) *Ling Shu or The Spiritual Pivot.* Hawaii: University of Hawaii Press.
19 Wang, Z. & Wang, J. (2007) *Ling Shu Acupuncture.* Irvine, CA: Ling Shu Press.

exterior and they act as a protective mechanism and buffer to hold pathogens. The classics indicate that the luo mai are at the superficial layer of the body and are treated with the prick-to-bleed method to release the pathogen(s). If they are not released, their pathogens can transfer to the main channels and the internal organs. The *Nei Jing* and the *Jia Yi Jing* support that the luo collaterals are located at the superficial areas of the body and are bled to release pathogens, and there is clear guidance that they cannot treat the internal organs.

The *Ling Shu* meticulously describes the function and symptoms of the main channels and distinguishes them from luo mai. That classic also recommends treatment plans that balance the main channels and the internal organs. Those treatment strategies include using the main channels, not the luo mai.

The basis of the transverse luo theory is a hypothesis that does not provide supporting acupuncture theory. Jizhou Yang's source-luo, host-guest acupuncture point combination from an unknown origin with no supporting acupuncture theory is the basis of this transverse luo channel hypothesis. NVN and others offer no explanation for the variance and direct conflict with the classical luo collateral theory and clinical application. The variance is significant as it treats the luo collaterals in a way that can drive pathogens deeper into the body and the internal organs, and it attempts to treat the luo points in ways the classics state it cannot treat: they treat the luo collateral network at the superficial level; they cannot treat at the bone (deep) level of the body.

The conclusion of this review is that the source-luo point combination and the transverse luo theory are not supported by acupuncture theory. The theories offer no explanation of the variance from the common use of the luo collaterals and luo points prior to the hypothesis and present no meaningful explanation of the risks in the treatment. Classical acupuncture offers guidance for treating the luo collaterals, as well as guidance for treating the main channels and organs.

There is a clarity and precision in the classical acupuncture channel system. There are five main channel systems: sinew channels, luo collaterals, main channels, divergent channels and the Eight Extraordinary Vessels. Using the entire channel system allows the practitioner to target the location of imbalances and be precise in treatment, which increases clinical effectiveness.

Conclusion

Chinese acupuncture has a long history with many theories, methods and techniques added over the past 2000 years. The style of writing and presentation from the Han dynasty to the current time lacks clarity in essential elements a practitioner needs to create acupuncture treatments and apply them in the clinic. *Clinical Point Selection* is my attempt to present a clear model for understanding how acupuncture works and how the practitioner can use that understanding to create acupuncture treatments—based on classical and traditional Chinese medical theories and applications, and my own insights.

Clinical Point Selection presents an approach for creating acupuncture treatments that can be combined with most traditions of acupuncture. It can also be a stand-alone system that can treat a high percentage of conditions found in a modern clinic. The theories, principles and framework in this book provide a flexible approach to creating acupuncture treatments, and the basis for customizing treatments for each person.

I hope you find this book beneficial in your clinical practice. Feel free to contact me about your experience applying the approaches in this book.

Best wishes,
David Twicken
July, 2024
The Year of the Dragon

Bibliography

Flaws, B. (2004) *The Classic of Difficulties: A Translation of the Nan Jing*. Boulder, CO: Blue Poppy Pressure.

Harper, D. (2007) *Early Chinese Medical Literature: The Mawangdui Medical Manuscripts*. London: Kegan Paul International.

Lu, H. (1985) *A Complete Translation of The Yellow Emperor's Classic of Internal Medicine and the Difficult Classic*. Vancouver: Academy of Oriental Heritage.

Maciocia, G. (2005) *The Foundations of Chinese Medicine: A Comprehensive Text for Acupuncturists and Herbalists*. Oxford: Churchill Livingstone.

Maciocia, G. (2006) *The Channels of Acupuncture: Clinical Use of the Secondary Channels and the Eight Extraordinary Vessels*. Oxford: Churchill Livingstone.

Matsumoto, K. & Birch, S. (1986) *Extraordinary Vessels*. Brookline, MA: Paradigm Publications.

McCann, H. (2014) *Pricking the Vessels: Blood Letting Therapy in Chinese Medicine*. London: Jessica Kingsley Publishers.

Morant, G.S. de (1972 French edition, 1994 English edition) *Chinese Acupuncture*. Chapter V. Brookline, MA: Paradigm Publications.

Ni, M. (1995) *The Yellow Emperor's Classic of Medicine: A New Translation of Neijing Suwen with Commentary*. Boston, MA: Shambhala.

Ni, Y. (1996) *Navigating the Channels of Traditional Chinese Medicine*. San Diego, CA: Complementary Medicine Press.

Twicken, D. (2011) *I Ching Acupuncture—The Balance Method: Clinical Applications of the Ba Gua and I Ching*. London: Singing Dragon.

Twicken, D. (2013) *Eight Extraordinary Channels—Qi Jing Ba Mai: A Handbook for Clinical Practice and Nei Dan Inner Meditation*. London: Singing Dragon.

Twicken, D. (2014) *The Divergent Channels—Jing Bie: A Handbook for Clinical Practice and Five Shen Nei Dan Inner Meditation*. London: Singing Dragon.

Twicken, D. (2015) *The Luo Collaterals—A Handbook for Clinical Practice and Treating Emotions and the Shen and The Six Healing Sounds*. London: Singing Dragon.

Twicken, D. (2023) *Taoist Nei Dan Inner Meditation: An Accessible Guide*. London: Singing Dragon.

Unschuld, P. (1986) *Nan-Ching: The Classic of Difficult Issues*. University of California Press.

Unschuld, P. (2016) *Huang Di Nei Jing Ling Shu: The Ancient Classic on Needle Therapy*. University of California Press.

Wang, Z. & Wang, J. (2007) *Ling Shu Acupuncture*. Irvine, CA: Ling Shu Press.

Wilcox, L. (2010) *The Great Compendium of Acupuncture and Moxibustion*. Volume V. Portland, OR: The Chinese Medicine Database.

Wu, J. (2002) *Ling Shu or The Spiritual Pivot*. Hawaii: University of Hawaii Press.

Wu, N. & Wu, A. (2002) *Yellow Emperor's Canon of Internal Medicine*. Beijing: China Science Technology Press.

Yang, C. (2004) *A Systematic Classic of Acupuncture and Moxibustion*. Boulder, CO: Blue Poppy Press.

Index

acupuncture
    description of 21
    therapeutic effect of 34
    treatment effects 35–6
acupuncture points
    description of 9
    difference from channels 27–8
    in Han dynasty 67–81
    unifying with channels 34–5
alternating sequence 92–3
Applied Channel Theory in Chinese Medicine (Wang Ju-Yi) 23

back shu points 71–3
Birch, S. 140

Canon of Pulse (Mai Jing) 71
Chamfrault, Albert 154, 157
channel combinations
    six-channel pairs 62–3
    Yin-Yang paired channels 61–3
channel selection
    channel combinations 60–3
    internal-pathway connection treatments 64–5
    needling sequence 60
    quotes on 59–60
    targeting treatment 65–6
    treatment types 65
channels
    correspondences systems 24–5

    difference from acupuncture points 27–8
    functions of 22–5
    movement in 24
    Qi in 52–4
    structure of 22
    system of 21–2
    unifying with acupuncture points 34–5
    working within 37–45
Chen, Chao 38
Chinese Acupuncture (Morant) 151, 152
Chinese medicine
    models of 31–3
    pain treatments 111–12
Classic of Difficulties see *Nei Jing*
completion sequence 94
correspondences, systems of 24–5

deficit conditions 87–9
destination in treatments 42, 86
direction-based treatments 43–5
divergent channels
    description of 28–9

eight extraordinary vessels (EV) 29–30, 132–45
eight flowing and pooling points 134–7
embryonic stem cells 52

emotional treatments
    approaches to 97–8
    five-Shen model 98,
        99–102, 103–10
    roughness of life 98–9
    treatment strategies 102–10
excess conditions 89–90

five-phases acupuncture
    points 47–8, 66, 77–81
five-Shen model 98, 99–102,
    103–10
Flaws, B. 78
Foundations of Chinese
    Medicine (Maciocia) 53
front mu points 73–4

Great Compendium (Jizhou Yang)
    147
Great Compendium of Acupuncture
    and Moxibustion, The (Jizhou
    Yang) 146, 148–9, 150, 151, 155
Guide of Acupuncture, The
    (Dou Hanqing) 146

Han dynasty acupuncture points
    back shu points 71–3
    five-phases acupuncture
        points 77–81
    front mu points 73–4
    Nan Ching 77–81
    source points 68–71
    transporting points 75–7
    wide and narrow
        acupuncture theories 68
Hanquing, Duo 133, 145, 146
herbal medicine 83

imbalance 9
internal-pathway connection
    treatments 64–5
ipsilateral sequence 91–2

Jia Yi Jing 24, 29, 71, 134, 160
Jizhou Yang 146, 147, 148–9,
    150, 151, 152, 157, 160

Li Can 151
Ling Shu 21, 24
    channel selection 59–60, 61, 63
    divergent channels 28
    eight extraordinary vessels
        29, 30, 147, 148
    emotional treatments
        97, 99, 101–2
    Han dynasty acupuncture
        points 68–9, 71–2, 73, 75
    luo mai 125, 128, 132, 145,
        153, 155–6, 158, 160
    main channels 55, 56
    Nei Jing channel system 24, 25,
        26
    organ treatments 94–5
    pain treatments 113, 115, 121
    Qi 49
    treatment effects 35
    treatment plans 37
Ling Shu Acupuncture
    (Wang and Wang) 159
luo mai
    colors 126–7
    excess and deficiency 128–31
    pathogenic factors 125–6
    quotes on 123–5
    seasons 127
    treatment of 131–2, 145–61

Maciocia, Giovanni 40, 53
Mai Jing 71
main channels
    acupuncture treatment in 56–7
    description of 27
    quotes on 55–6
Matsumoto, K. 140
Mawangdui Silk Texts 17
meridians see channels
Morant, George Soulié
    De 151–3, 155, 157–9
mu points 73–5
musculoskeletal system 114–18

Nan Ching 10, 28, 47, 68,
    69, 70, 76, 77–81

INDEX

needling
    channel selection 60
    Han dynasty acupuncture
        points 70–1
    reducing/reinforcing
        technique 39–40
    sequence of 33–4
nei dan 41
Nei Jing 26, 28
    destination in treatments 41
    divergent channels 29
    eight extraordinary vessels 134
    emotional treatments 97, 105–6
    Han dynasty acupuncture
        points 67, 68–9, 70, 73, 75, 76
    luo mai 123–4, 160
    main channels 56
    needling 39–40
    pain treatments 114
    working within channels 37
Nei Jing channel system (Jing Luo)
    luo collaterals 26–7
    sinew channels 25–6
Nei Jing Ling Shu 17–19, 67
Nguyen Van Nghi (NVN)
    154, 155, 157, 158, 160
Ni, M. 42, 73, 125, 154

organ treatments
    alternating sequence 92–3
    completion sequence 94
    deficit conditions 87–9
    destination point 86
    excess conditions 89–90
    framework for 84–5
    goal of 83–4
    ipsilateral sequence 91–2
    herbal medicine 83
    Ling Shu spring-stream
        points treatment 94–5
    treatment sequence 85–6
    treatment strategies 90–1

pain treatments
    Chinese medicine 111–12
    musculoskeletal system 114–18

treatment plan 112
treatment principles 113–14
twelve-point theory 118–22
pathways *see* channels
Prescriptions Worth a Thousand
    Gold for Emergencies 71
primary channels *see* main channels
Pulse Classic (Jing Ming) 71

Qi
    in channels 52–4
    description of 10
    embryonic stem cells 52
    reducing/reinforcing
        technique in 49–54

reducing technique
    common teachings 48–9
    description of 9–10
    five-phases theory 47–8
    needling 39–40
    Qi 49–54
    working within channels 43
reinforcing technique
    common teachings 48–9
    description of 9–10
    five-phases theory 47–8
    needling 39–40
    Qi 49–54
    working within channels 42–3
Renying-Cunkou pulse
    19, 55, 61, 147, 148
Robertson, J. 23, 39

Shang Hang Lun (SHL) 83

shu points 71–3
sinew channels 25–6
six-channel pairs 62–3
source points 68–71
Su Wen 17, 24
    destination in treatments 42
    eight extraordinary vessels 29, 30
    emotional treatments 97, 99
    luo mai 124–5, 154, 155
    main channels 55–6

Su Wen cont.
    mu points 73
    Nei Jing channel system 26
    pain treatments 113, 115, 121
    working within channels 37

transporting points 75-7
twelve-point theory 118-22

Unschuld, P. 19, 50, 69, 70, 115, 156

Wang, J. 23, 28, 40, 55,
    75, 131, 138, 159
Wang, Z. 40, 55, 75, 131, 138, 159
Wilcox, L. 150
working within channels
    activity during treatment 38-9
    destination in treatments 42

direction-based treatments 43-5
needling method 39-40
nei dan 41
reducing technique 43
reinforcing technique 42-3
Wu, A. 42, 113
Wu, J. 13, 37, 39, 69, 71, 102,
    113, 115, 131, 132, 156, 159
Wu, N. 42, 113
Wu Xing 75-7

Yang, C. 29, 74
Yin-Yang paired channels 61-3
Yixue Rumen (Li Can) 151

zangfu 31, 49-50, 53-4, 68, 76
Zhen Jiu Da Cheng (Jizhou Yang)
    146, 148-9, 150, 151, 155